Communications in Computer and Information Science 2079

Editorial Board Members

Joaquim Filipe ⓘ, *Polytechnic Institute of Setúbal, Setúbal, Portugal*
Ashish Ghosh ⓘ, *Indian Statistical Institute, Kolkata, India*
Lizhu Zhou, *Tsinghua University, Beijing, China*

Rationale

The CCIS series is devoted to the publication of proceedings of computer science conferences. Its aim is to efficiently disseminate original research results in informatics in printed and electronic form. While the focus is on publication of peer-reviewed full papers presenting mature work, inclusion of reviewed short papers reporting on work in progress is welcome, too. Besides globally relevant meetings with internationally representative program committees guaranteeing a strict peer-reviewing and paper selection process, conferences run by societies or of high regional or national relevance are also considered for publication.

Topics

The topical scope of CCIS spans the entire spectrum of informatics ranging from foundational topics in the theory of computing to information and communications science and technology and a broad variety of interdisciplinary application fields.

Information for Volume Editors and Authors

Publication in CCIS is free of charge. No royalties are paid, however, we offer registered conference participants temporary free access to the online version of the conference proceedings on SpringerLink (http://link.springer.com) by means of an http referrer from the conference website and/or a number of complimentary printed copies, as specified in the official acceptance email of the event.

CCIS proceedings can be published in time for distribution at conferences or as post-proceedings, and delivered in the form of printed books and/or electronically as USBs and/or e-content licenses for accessing proceedings at SpringerLink. Furthermore, CCIS proceedings are included in the CCIS electronic book series hosted in the SpringerLink digital library at http://link.springer.com/bookseries/7899. Conferences publishing in CCIS are allowed to use Online Conference Service (OCS) for managing the whole proceedings lifecycle (from submission and reviewing to preparing for publication) free of charge.

Publication process

The language of publication is exclusively English. Authors publishing in CCIS have to sign the Springer CCIS copyright transfer form, however, they are free to use their material published in CCIS for substantially changed, more elaborate subsequent publications elsewhere. For the preparation of the camera-ready papers/files, authors have to strictly adhere to the Springer CCIS Authors' Instructions and are strongly encouraged to use the CCIS LaTeX style files or templates.

Abstracting/Indexing

CCIS is abstracted/indexed in DBLP, Google Scholar, EI-Compendex, Mathematical Reviews, SCImago, Scopus. CCIS volumes are also submitted for the inclusion in ISI Proceedings.

How to start

To start the evaluation of your proposal for inclusion in the CCIS series, please send an e-mail to ccis@springer.com.

Ana Moita · Katja Bühler · Hesham Ali ·
Ning Deng · Ioanna Chouvarda ·
Federico Cabitza · Ana Fred · Hugo Gamboa
Editors

Biomedical Engineering Systems and Technologies

16th International Joint Conference, BIOSTEC 2023
Lisbon, Portugal, February 16–18, 2023
Revised Selected Papers

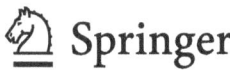

Editors
Ana Moita
Instituto Superior Técnico
Lisbon, Portugal

Hesham Ali
University of Nebraska at Omaha
Omaha, NE, USA

Ioanna Chouvarda
Aristotle University of Thessaloniki
Thessaloniki, Greece

Ana Fred
Instituto Superior Técnico
Lisbon, Portugal

Instituto de Telecomunicações
Lisbon, Portugal

Katja Bühler
VRVis Zentrum für Virtual Reality und
Visualisierung Forschungs-GmbH
Vienna, Austria

Ning Deng
Zhejiang University
Zhejiang, China

Federico Cabitza
Università degli Studi di Milano-Bicocca
Milan, Italy

Hugo Gamboa
Nova University of Lisbon
Caparica, Portugal

ISSN 1865-0929   ISSN 1865-0937 (electronic)
Communications in Computer and Information Science
ISBN 978-3-031-67087-9   ISBN 978-3-031-67088-6 (eBook)
https://doi.org/10.1007/978-3-031-67088-6

© The Editor(s) (if applicable) and The Author(s), under exclusive license
to Springer Nature Switzerland AG 2024

This work is subject to copyright. All rights are solely and exclusively licensed by the Publisher, whether the whole or part of the material is concerned, specifically the rights of translation, reprinting, reuse of illustrations, recitation, broadcasting, reproduction on microfilms or in any other physical way, and transmission or information storage and retrieval, electronic adaptation, computer software, or by similar or dissimilar methodology now known or hereafter developed.
The use of general descriptive names, registered names, trademarks, service marks, etc. in this publication does not imply, even in the absence of a specific statement, that such names are exempt from the relevant protective laws and regulations and therefore free for general use.
The publisher, the authors and the editors are safe to assume that the advice and information in this book are believed to be true and accurate at the date of publication. Neither the publisher nor the authors or the editors give a warranty, expressed or implied, with respect to the material contained herein or for any errors or omissions that may have been made. The publisher remains neutral with regard to jurisdictional claims in published maps and institutional affiliations.

This Springer imprint is published by the registered company Springer Nature Switzerland AG
The registered company address is: Gewerbestrasse 11, 6330 Cham, Switzerland

If disposing of this product, please recycle the paper.

Preface

We are excited to present this book that includes revised and extended versions of a set of selected research papers that were presented at the 16th International Joint Conference on Biomedical Engineering Systems and Technologies (BIOSTEC 2023), held in Lisbon, Portugal, from 16–18 February.

BIOSTEC is a unique event that is composed of co-located conferences that represent five key knowledge areas related to Biomedical Informatics. They are HEALTHINF, BIOINFORMATICS, BIOSIGNALS, BIODEVICES and BIOIMAGING. Collectively, the five conferences of BIOSTEC 2023 received 246 paper submissions from 45 countries, of which 3% were included in this book.

The papers were selected by the chairs of each conference. The selection was based on several academic criteria including the review reports and comments provided by the program committee members, the session chairs' assessment of the presentations, and the program chairs' global view of all papers included in the technical program. The authors of the selected papers were then invited to submit revised and extended versions of their papers that include at least 30% additional innovative material.

The main objective of the joint BIOSTEC conferences is to bring together researchers and practitioners, including engineers, biologists, health professionals and informatics/computer scientists, to meet and discuss the recent trends and innovations in various aspects related to Biomedical Informatics. Over the years, this event has attracted diverse groups of participants interested in both theoretical advances and applications of information systems, artificial intelligence, signal processing, electronics and other engineering tools in knowledge areas related to biosciences and healthcare.

The papers selected to be included in this publication contribute to the understanding of relevant trends of current research on Biomedical Engineering Systems and Technologies that include Pattern Recognition and Machine Learning, Decision Support Systems, Data Mining and Data Analysis, eHealth Applications, eHealth, Detection and Identification, Computational Intelligence, Cognitive Informatics, Big Data in Healthcare and Assistive Technologies.

The success of the BIOSTEC conferences and their subsequent publications would not have been possible without the support of several dedicated and enthusiastic groups.

We would like to thank all the authors for their contributions as well as the session chairs and the reviewers who have helped to ensure the quality of this publication.

February 2023

Ana Moita
Katja Bühler
Hesham Ali
Ning Deng
Ioanna Chouvarda
Federico Cabitza
Ana Fred
Hugo Gamboa

Organization

Conference Co-chairs

BIOSTEC

Ana Fred	University of Lisbon, Portugal
Hugo Gamboa	Nova University of Lisbon, Portugal

Program Co-chairs

BIODEVICES

Ana Moita — University of Lisbon and Academia Militar, Portugal

BIOIMAGING

Katja Bühler — VRVis, Austria

BIOINFORMATICS

Hesham Ali	University of Nebraska at Omaha, USA
Ning Deng	Zhejiang University, China

BIOSIGNALS

Ioanna Chouvarda — Aristotle University of Thessaloniki, Greece

HEALTHINF

Federico Cabitza — Università degli Studi di Milano-Bicocca and IRCCS Ospedale Galeazzi, Italy

Program Committee

BIODEVICES

Carlos Abreu	Instituto Politécnico de Viana do Castelo, Portugal
Paulo Antunes	Aveiro University and i3N, Portugal
Steve Beeby	University of Southampton, UK
Vanessa Cardoso	University of Minho, Portugal
Eric Chappel	Debiotech SA, Switzerland
Mostafa Charmi	University of Zanjan, Iran
Cheng-Hsin Chuang	National Sun Yat-sen University, Taiwan, Republic of China
Youngjae Chun	University of Pittsburgh, USA
Alberto Cliquet Jr.	University of São Paulo & University of Campinas, Brazil
Maria Evelina Fantacci	University of Pisa and INFN, Italy
Mireya Fernández Chimeno	Universitat Politècnica de Catalunya, Spain
Francisco Gamiz	University of Granada, Spain
Miguel García Gonzalez	Universitat Politècnica de Catalunya, Spain
Javier Garcia-Casado	Universitat Politècnica de València, Spain
Gianluca Gatti	University of Calabria, Italy
Fernanda Irrera	University of Rome "Sapienza", Italy
Dean Krusienski	Virginia Commonwealth University, USA
Hiroshi Kumagai	Kitasato University, Japan
Dumitru Mazilu	National Institutes of Health and Human Services, USA
Simona Miclaus	Nicolae Balcescu Land Forces Academy, Romania
Robert Newcomb	University of Maryland, USA
Abraham Otero	Universidad San Pablo CEU, Spain
Helena Pereira	Coimbra Institute for Biomedical Imaging and Translational Research, Portugal
Wim Rutten	University of Twente, Netherlands
Seonghan Ryu	Hannam University, Korea, Republic of
Michael Schöning	FH Aachen, Germany
Mauro Serpelloni	University of Brescia, Italy
Giuseppe Tronci	University of Leeds, UK
John Tudor	University of Southampton, UK
Pankaj Vadgama	Queen Mary University of London, UK
Duarte Valério	Universidade de Lisboa, Portugal
Renato Varoto	Independent Researcher, Brazil

Additional Reviewers

BIODEVICES

Dogangun Uzun	National Heart, Lung, and Blood Institute, National Institutes of Health, USA

Program Committee

BIOIMAGING

Peter Balazs	University of Szeged, Hungary
Richard Bayford	Middlesex University London, UK
Alpan Bek	Middle East Technical University, Turkey
Heang-Ping Chan	University of Michigan, USA
Mostafa Charmi	University of Zanjan, Iran
Miguel Coimbra	University of Porto, Portugal
Costel Flueraru	National Research Council of Canada, Canada
Carlos Geraldes	Universidade de Coimbra, Portugal
Dimitris Gorpas	Technical University of Munich, Germany
Tzung-Pei Hong	National University of Kaohsiung, Taiwan, Republic of China
Jae Youn Hwang	DGIST, Korea, Republic of
Algimantas Krisciukaitis	Lithuanian University of Health Sciences, Lithuania
Hongen Liao	Tsinghua University, China
Lucia Maddalena	ICAR, National Research Council (CNR), Italy
Kunal Mitra	Florida Institute of Technology, USA
Joanna Isabelle Olszewska	University of the West of Scotland, UK
Kalman Palagyi	University of Szeged, Hungary
Vadim Perez	Instituto Mexicano del Seguro Social, Mexico
Gregory Sharp	Massachusetts General Hospital, USA
Leonid Shvartsman	Hebrew University, Israel
Arkadiusz Tomczyk	Lodz University of Technology, Poland
Carlos Travieso-González	Universidad de Las Palmas de Gran Canaria, Spain
Benjamin Tsui	Johns Hopkins University, USA
Vladimír Ulman	Masaryk University, Czech Republic

Jing Wang   University of Texas Southwestern Medical
                                  Center, USA
Yuanyuan Wang   Fudan University, China

Program Committee

BIOINFORMATICS

Mohamed Abouelhoda   Nile University, Egypt
Heba Afify   Cairo University, Egypt
Tatsuya Akutsu   Kyoto University, Japan
Payam Behzadi   Shahr-e-Qods Branch, Islamic Azad University,
                                  Iran
Gilles Bernot   Université Côte d'Azur, France
Stefano Calza   University of Brescia, Italy
Jean-Paul Comet   Université Côte d'Azur, France
Keith Crandall   George Washington University, USA
Thomas Dandekar   University of Würzburg, Germany
Maria Evelina Fantacci   University of Pisa and INFN, Italy
Alexandru Floares   SAIA, Romania
Dmitrij Frishman   Technical University of Munich, Germany
Junguk Hur   University of North Dakota School of Medicine
                                  and Health Sciences, USA
Giuseppe Jurman   Fondazione Bruno Kessler, Italy
Jirí Kléma   Czech Technical University in Prague, Czech
                                  Republic
Ivan Kulakovskiy   IPR RAS, Russian Federation
Man-Kee Lam   Universiti Teknologi PETRONAS, Malaysia
Carlile Lavor   University of Campinas, Brazil
Enzo Martegani   University of Milano-Bicocca, Italy
Paolo Milazzo   Università di Pisa, Italy
Jason Miller   Shepherd University, USA
José Molina   Universidad Carlos III de Madrid, Spain
Javier Reina-Tosina   University of Seville, Spain
Laura Roa   University of Seville, Spain
Vincent Rodin   UBO, LabSTICC/CNRS, France
Ulrich Rückert   Bielefeld University, Germany
J. Cristian Salgado   University of Chile, Chile
Andrew Schumann   University of Information Technology and
                                  Management in Rzeszow, Poland
João Setubal   Universidade de São Paulo, Brazil

Sylvain Soliman	Inria Saclay, France
Peter Sykacek	University of Natural Resources and Life Sciences, Vienna, Austria
Y-H. Taguchi	Chuo University, Japan
Giorgio Valentini	University of Milan, Italy

Additional Reviewers

BIOINFORMATICS

Artem Kasianov	IITP RAS, Russian Federation
Pavel Kravchenko	Max Planck Institute of Biochemistry, Germany

Program Committee

BIOSIGNALS

Eda Akman Aydin	Gazi University, Turkey
Raul Alcaraz	University of Castilla-La Mancha, Spain
Robert Allen	University of Southampton, UK
Eberhard Beck	Brandenburg University of Applied Sciences, Germany
Maria Claudia Castro	Centro Universitário FEI, Brazil
Adam Czajka	University of Notre Dame, USA
Petr Dolezel	University of Pardubice, Czech Republic
Seraina Dual	KTH Royal Institute of Technology, Sweden
Dimitris Filos	Aristotle University of Thessaloniki, Greece
Javier Garcia-Casado	Universitat Politècnica de València, Spain
Pedro Gómez Vilda	Independent Researcher, Spain
Inan Güler	Gazi University, Turkey
Thomas Hinze	Friedrich Schiller University Jena, Germany
Roberto Hornero	University of Valladolid, Spain
Jiri Jan	Brno University of Technology, Czech Republic
Aleksandar Jeremic	McMaster University, Canada
Akos Jobbagy	Budapest Univ. of Tech. and Econ., Hungary
Gordana Jovanovic Dolecek	Institute INAOE, Mexico
Natalya Kizilova	Warsaw University of Technology, Poland
Krzysztof Kulpa	Independent Researcher, Poland

Lenka Lhotska	Czech Technical University in Prague, Czech Republic
Harald Loose	Brandenburg University of Applied Sciences, Germany
Luca Mainardi	Politecnico di Milano, Italy
Fernando Monteiro	Polytechnic Institute of Bragança, Portugal
Mihaela Morega	University Politehnica of Bucharest, Romania
Minoru Nakayama	Tokyo Institute of Technology, Japan
Joanna Isabelle Olszewska	University of the West of Scotland, UK
Rui Pedro Paiva	University of Coimbra, Portugal
Vasileios Papapanagiotou	Aristotle University of Thessaloniki, Greece
Riccardo Pernice	University of Palermo, Italy
Vitor Pires	Instituto Politécnico de Setúbal, Portugal
Fabienne Poree	Université de Rennes, France
Shitala Prasad	I2R, A*Star, Singapore
José Joaquín Rieta	Universidad Politécnica de Valencia, Spain
Heather Ruskin	Dublin City University, Ireland
Giovanni Saggio	Tor Vergata University of Rome, Italy
Andrews Samraj	Mahendra Engineering College, India
Reinhard Schneider	Fachhochschule Vorarlberg, Austria
Lotfi Senhadji	University of Rennes 1, France
Zdenek Smekal	Brno University of Technology, Czech Republic
Jordi Solé-Casals	University of Vic - Central University of Catalonia, Spain
António Teixeira	University of Aveiro, Portugal
Carlos Thomaz	Centro Universitário FEI, Brazil
Hua-Nong Ting	University of Malaya, Malaysia
Carlos Travieso-González	Universidad de Las Palmas de Gran Canaria, Spain
Pedro Vaz	University of Coimbra, Portugal
Yuanyuan Wang	Fudan University, China
Rafal Zdunek	Politechnika Wrocławska, Poland

Additional Reviewers

BIOSIGNALS

Ana Rocha	University of Aveiro, Portugal
Ioannis Sarafis	Aristotle University of Thessaloniki, Greece

Program Committee

HEALTHINF

Carlos Abreu	Instituto Politécnico de Viana do Castelo, Portugal
Luca Anselma	Università degli Studi di Torino, Italy
Gabriella Balestra	Politecnico di Torino, Italy
Payam Behzadi	Shahr-e-Qods Branch, Islamic Azad University, Iran
José Alberto Benítez-Andrades	Universidad de León, Spain
Sorana Bolboaca	Iuliu Hatieganu University of Medicine and Pharmacy, Cluj-Napoca, Romania
Silvia Bonfanti	University of Bergamo, Italy
Alessio Bottrighi	Università del Piemonte Orientale, Italy
Frederico Branco	University of Trás-os-Montes e Alto Douro, Portugal
Klaus Brinker	Hamm-Lippstadt University of Applied Sciences, Germany
Andrea Campagner	University of Milano-Bicocca, Italy
Malcolm Clarke	Ondokuz Mayis University, Turkey
Mihail Cocosila	Athabasca University, Canada
Emmanuel Conchon	XLIM, France
George Drosatos	Athena Research Center, Greece
Gilles Falquet	University of Geneva, Switzerland
Daniela Fogli	Università degli Studi di Brescia, Italy
Christoph Friedrich	Dortmund University of Applied Sciences and Arts, Germany
Sebastian Fudickar	University of Lübeck, Germany
Henry Gabb	Intel Corporation, USA
Angelo Gargantini	University of Bergamo, Italy
David Greenhalgh	University of Strathclyde, UK
Frank Harmsen	Maastricht University, Netherlands
Dragan Jankovic	University of Niš, Serbia
Dimitrios Katehakis	FORTH, Greece
Josef Kohout	University of West Bohemia, Czech Republic
Haridimos Kondylakis	Foundation for Research and Technology - Hellas, Greece
Tomohiro Kuroda	Kyoto University Hospital, Japan
Erwin Lemche	King's College London, UK
Lenka Lhotska	Czech Technical University in Prague, Czech Republic
Guillaume Lopez	Aoyama Gakuin University, Japan

Martin Lopez-Nores	University of Vigo, Spain
Constantinos Loukas	National and Kapodistrian University of Athens, Greece
Chi-Jie Lu	Fu Jen Catholic University, Taiwan, Republic of China
Gang Luo	University of Washington, USA
Alda Marques	University of Aveiro, Portugal
Juan Martinez-Romo	National University of Distance Education, Spain
Ken Masters	Sultan Qaboos University, Oman
Vincenzo Mea	University of Udine, Italy
Stefania Montani	Piemonte Orientale University, Italy
Alberto Morán	Universidad Autónoma de Baja California, Mexico
Roman Moucek	University of West Bohemia, Czech Republic
Nelson Pacheco da Rocha	University of Aveiro, Portugal
Alessandro Pagano	University of Bari, Italy
Marco Painho	Nova Information Management School, Portugal
Rui Pedro Paiva	University of Coimbra, Portugal
Hugo Paredes	INESC TEC and University of Tras-os-Montes e Alto Douro, Portugal
Antonio Piccinno	University of Bari, Italy
Mahmudur Rahman	Morgan State University, USA
Arkalgud Ramaprasad	University of Illinois at Chicago, USA
Grzegorz Redlarski	Gdańsk University of Technology, Poland
Alejandro Rodríguez González	Centro de Tecnología Biomédica, Spain
Cristian Rotariu	Grigore T. Popa University of Medicine and Pharmacy, Romania
George Sakellaropoulos	University of Patras, Greece
Hashem Salarzadeh Jenatabadi	University of Malaya, Malaysia
Ovidio Salvetti	National Research Council of Italy - CNR, Italy
Akio Sashima	AIST, Japan
Bettina Schnor	University of Potsdam, Germany
Daniel Schulman	Philips Research North America, USA
Carla Simone	University of Milano-Bicocca, Italy
Åsa Smedberg	Stockholm University, Sweden
Francesco Tiezzi	University of Camerino, Italy
Marie Travers	University of Limerick, Ireland
Yi-Ju Tseng	National Yang Ming Chiao Tung University, Taiwan, Republic of China
Lauri Tuovinen	University of Oulu, Finland
Mohy Uddin	King Abdullah International Medical Research Center, Saudi Arabia
Gary Ushaw	Newcastle University, UK

Sitalakshmi Venkatraman	Melbourne Polytechnic, Australia
Francisco Veredas	Universidad de Málaga, Spain
Chien-Chih Wang	Ming Chi University of Technology, Taiwan, Republic of China
Dimitrios Zarakovitis	University of the Peloponnese, Greece

Additional Reviewers

HEALTHINF

Olivier Blazy	École Polytechnique, France

Invited Speakers

BIOSTEC

Giovanni Saggio	Tor Vergata University of Rome, Italy
Elazer Edelman	Massachusetts Institute of Technology, USA
Mireille Hildebrandt	Vrije Universiteit Brussel, Belgium
Riccardo Bellazzi	Università di Pavia, Italy

Contents

Towards Robust Homography Estimation for Forward-Motion Panorama
for Multi-camera Wireless Capsule Endoscopy Videos 1
   Marina Oliveira and Helder Araujo

Estimation of Fluid Intake Volume from Surface Electromyography
Signals: A Comparative Study Between Subject-Specific and Global
Regression Techniques 24
   Iman A. Ismail and Ernest N. Kamavuako

Epileptic Seizure Detection and Prediction for Patient Support 40
   *Gul Hameed Khan, Nadeem Ahmad Khan, Wala Saadeh,
and Muahammad Awais Bin Altaf*

Topic Modelling and Interpretable Cost Estimation for Medical Insurance
Fraud Detection 60
   James Kemp, Christopher Barker, Norm Good, and Michael Bain

Improving Patient Trajectory Forecasts in Hospitals: Using Emergency
Department Data for Length of Stay Prediction and Next Hospital Unit
Classification 84
   Alexander Winter, Toralf Kirsten, and Mattis Hartwig

Suroy-Suroy: An Immersive Virtual Reality Therapy Game for Persons
Living with Dementia in the Philippines 107
   *Veeda Michelle M. Anlacan, Angelo Cedric F. Panganiban,
Roland Dominic G. Jamora, Isabel Teresa O. Salido,
Romuel Aloizeus Z. Apuya, Bryan Andrei C. Galecio, Michael L. Tee,
Maria Eliza R. Aguila, Cherica A. Tee, and Jaime D. L. Caro*

The Impact of Feature Selection on Balancing, Based on Diabetes Data 125
   Diogo Machado, Vítor Santos Costa, and Pedro Brandão

Author Index 147

Towards Robust Homography Estimation for Forward-Motion Panorama for Multi-camera Wireless Capsule Endoscopy Videos

Marina Oliveira(✉) and Helder Araujo

Institute of Systems and Robotics, Department of Electrical and Computer Engineering, Faculty of Sciences and Technology, 3004-531 Coimbra, Portugal
marina.oliveira@student.uc.pt

Abstract. A noteworthy challenge in Wireless Capsule Endoscopy is the significant time and expertise required by medical professionals to accurately interpret its videos and detect anomalies. The combination of a large number of frames to analyze within each video coupled with poor image quality contributes to low lesion detection rates. To address these issues, our study explores a methodology for the construction of local forward and/or backward-motion panoramic overviews from videos rendered from a synthetic tubular model created in Blender. This approach aims to consolidate essential information from multiple frames for the purpose of lesion detection and localization. The mosaicing process is explored by computing global homographies between sequential frames and three methods for homography estimation are assessed. This study compares the resulting local panoramas obtained with our method with those produced using a deep neural network approach, utilizing three different models for image quality assessment.

Keywords: Capsule movement · Deep learning · Feature-extraction · panorama · Optical flow · Wireless capsule endoscopy

1 Introduction

The configuration for a Wireless Capsule Endoscopy (WCE) procedure comprises a capsule with one or more miniaturized cameras, a light source, and a wireless transmission circuit. Following ingestion, the capsule traverses the GI tract, driven by peristalsis, leading to an unpredictable motion pattern. Each capsule is equipped with light-emitting diodes and one or more cameras that feature a fixed or an adjustable frame rate. The frames are then transmitted to a recording device for review by a healthcare professional [5].

There are several commercially available capsules for examinations of the GI tract, with wireless and non-wireless transmission circuits. From Fig. 1, PillCam SB and SB2

Supported by Institute of Systems and Robotics, from University of Coimbra, Portugal.

© The Author(s), under exclusive license to Springer Nature Switzerland AG 2024
A. Moita et al. (Eds.): BIOSTEC 2023, CCIS 2079, pp. 1–23, 2024.
https://doi.org/10.1007/978-3-031-67088-6_1

are older versions and are no longer commercially available. SB3 is the most recent version for small bowel inspection. PillCam SB3 is a single-lens camera capsule with a field of view of 172° and an adaptive frame rate of 2 to 6 images per second based on the capsule movement. For colon inspection, the currently available capsule is the PillCam COLON2. PillCam Crohn's is also currently commercially available. PillCam Crohn's and PillCam COLON2 both have a dual-lens camera capsule with a field of view of 172° per camera and an adaptive frame rate of 4 to 35 frames per second based on the speed of the capsule. The capsules shown in Fig. 2 are currently commercially available.

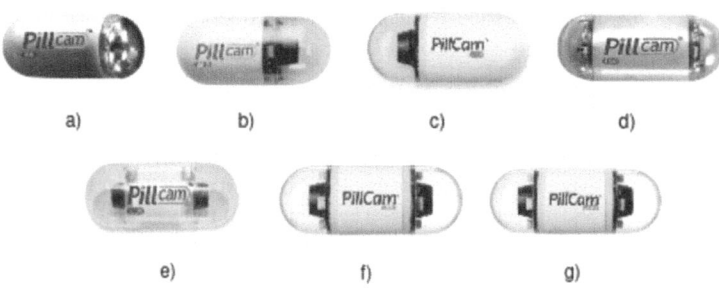

Fig. 1. PillCam camera capsules from Medtronic: a) PillCam SB (Small Bowell); b) PillCam SB2; c) PillCam SB3; d) PillCam ESO (Esophagus); e) PillCam COLON; f) PillCam COLON2; g) PillCam Crohn's (Adapted from [4]).

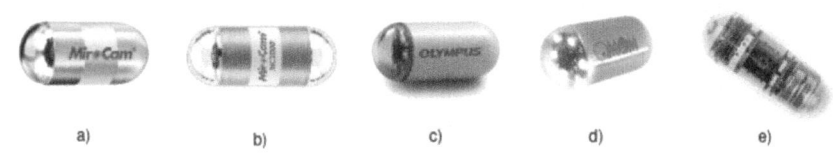

Fig. 2. Other camera capsules: a) MiroCam from Intromedic; b) Mirocam MC2000 from Intromedic; c) EndoCapsule from Olympus; d) OMOM from Jinshan; e) CapsoCam Plus from CapsoVision. (Adapted from [4]).

An eight-hour WCE video normally comprises approximately 50,000 frames [20]. The screening process using specific software demands several hours of focused attention from clinicians to identify, differentiate, and pinpoint a broad range of gastrointestinal (GI) lesions, such as the ones illustrated in Fig. 3, throughout the GI tract. A significant limitation that can lower detection rates to 40% is the poor quality of the frames [20]. Strategies that aim to reduce viewing time and improve detection rates focus on the selection of the most representative frames (MRF) within ach video. Tools like the RAPID Reader software enable simultaneous screening of multiple frames. The

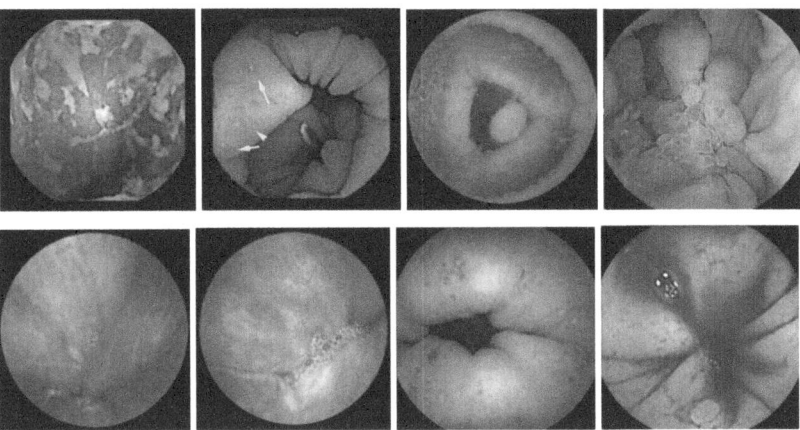

Fig. 3. Sample of WCE frames that represent examples of the most frequent lesions that can be identified in the gastrointestinal tract, especially in the area of the small bowell. The first four images correspond to (from left to right): Ulcerative Colitis, Chron's Disease Ulcer, Polyp and Tumor-Mass. The second set of images correspond to (from left to right): Melanosis Coli, Hemorrhoids, Erosions and Bleeding. (Adapted from the Atlas of the PillCam Rapid Reader Software [15])

QuickView algorithm enhances efficiency by adjusting frame rates in stable regions and stabilizing them in sequences with abrupt changes [20]. Other summarization techniques can condense videos by up to 90% by creating epitomes from clusters of frames containing previously identified anomalies [8].

A reduced field of view is another factor that lowers detection rates [21]. The viewing angle, determined by the light passing through the camera lens [23], is essential for a comprehensive examination. The commercially available capsules previously mentioned typically feature cameras with viewing angles ranging from 140 to 170° [2]. Capsules that incorporate multiple cameras, such as two cameras positioned at opposite ends of the capsule aim to address this limitation.

1.1 Panorama Construction

To broaden the field of view and increase the area of analysis without any hardware alteration, approaches exploring the construction of panoramic views of local regions of interest would be a valuable solution, taking advantage of the fact that each cameras from same capsule captures the same tissue structures. A full-trajectory panorama or multiple local panoramas in certain regions of interest would provide a summarized overview of the WCE videos, lower viewing time and improving detection rates.

A full panorama construction implicates a thorough surface geometry reconstruction and the associated estimation of motion [24]. The chosen procedure may differ depending on how the sequential frames are captured since it defines the geometry of the problem [3].

For a panoramic view computation, each dataset can be obtained with:

1. **a single camera** that ideally undergoes **pure rotation** around a known optical axis;
2. **multiple cameras**, resulting in frames with overlapping domains;
3. **one or more cameras** that move ideally with **pure translation** along the known optical axis, as shown in Fig. 4a).
4. **one or more cameras** that move with **rotation and translation** along the known optical axis, as shown in Fig. 4c).
5. **one or more cameras** that move with **rotation and translation** along an axis that does not coincide with the optical axis, as shown in Fig. 4d).

In the case of Fig. 4b), where **one or more cameras** move ideally with **pure rotation** around the known optical axis, there is no new information between sequential frames, so there is no possible panorama. In cases 3)–5), the goal is to recognise overlapping radial domains from each set of sequential frames and stitch them to obtain a forward or backward-motion mosaic [3].

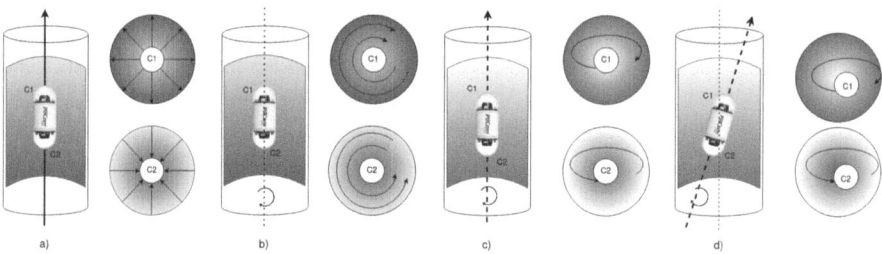

Fig. 4. Capsule-motion possibilities inside the GI tract (in this case a PillCam Colon2 double-camera wireless capsule): a) one or more cameras that move ideally with pure translation along the known optical axis; b) one or more cameras move ideally with pure rotation around the known optical axis; c) one or more cameras that move with rotation and translation along the known optical axis; d) one or more cameras that move with rotation and translation along an axis that does not coincide with the optical axis [15].

Our methodology intends to overcome the above-mentioned limitations through the construction of forward or backward-motion local panoramas. We present the steps towards a solution that aims to take into account both the geometry of the problem and the particularities that come with working with WCE videos.

With medical images, mosaicing processes have many challenges since the different tissues have various appearances, so feature-extraction procedures are hard to generalise. The registration of the same scene from different views is a challenge in itself since the deformation of the tissue is non-rigid and the images are prone to specular reflections. The illumination is non-homogeneous since the light source is within the capsule itself that moves along the GI tract and the path can occasionally be blocked by blood and/or other artefacts. A significant challenge is the estimation of a transformation that robustly maps the different views into a single mosaic with an interpolation algorithm that smoothly blends the pixel intensities so that the result can be clinically interpretative [11].

1.2 Image Registration

Image Registration approaches can be direct pixel-based and feature-based. The **Scale-Invariant Feature Transform (SIFT)** algorithm detects stable points in the scale space using a cascade filtering procedure. Keypoint descriptors are created from local geometric deformations represented by blurred difference of Gaussians (DoG) image gradients in various orientation planes at multiple scales and compared with each new frame. The points that minimize the Euclidean distance between feature vectors are selected. A final subset of matches is assigned based on position, scale, and orientation. The SIFT features are partially invariant to illumination changes and distortion, resistant to image noise, and remain invariant to scaling, rotation, and translation [16].

Optical-flow (OF) based registration is less common, especially with deep learning. OF measures the displacement between two images based on image intensity. OF can be computed with gradient-based (GB) methods, which may degenerate the computation due to specularities, matching-based methods that interpolate flow field for each pixel, and energy minimization methods that use dense information from the whole frame but can be affected by inconsistent specular reflections [11].

Generalized Pipe Representation. To transform the radial displacement of image pixels into parallel displacement, a 2D planar image is projected onto a 3D cylinder using pipe projection. The axis of the pipe $s = S/|S|$ passes through the optical center $O = (0,0,0)$ and the focus of expansion (FOE) $S = (s_x, s_y, f_c)$, with f_c as the focal length. Each point Q is the projection of each original point $P = (x, y, f_c)$, distanced from the axis s by the radius R of the pipe, and collinear with both P and O. The 3D position of a point Q on the pipe is expressed in Eq. (1) [15, 17].

$$Q = (Q_x, Q_y, Q_z) = k\hat{s} + Rcos(\alpha)\hat{d} + Rsin(\alpha)\hat{r} \qquad (1)$$

with k as the position along the axis $\hat{s}$, with $\hat{d}$ and $\hat{r}$ as unit vectors chosen to form a cartesian coordinate system together with $\hat{s}$ and α as the angle from $\hat{d}$. To preserve the geometry and resolution of the image, the radius of the pipe projection is selected as $R = \sqrt{f_c^2 + (\frac{w}{2})^2 + (\frac{h}{2})^2}$, where w is the width and h is the height of the image. The resolution decreases as $|Q_z - f_c|$, so it is best preserved around the intersection of the pipe with the image plane ($Q_z = f_c$) [15, 17].

Pipe Mosaicing. The flow vector (u,v) between two corresponding points $P_k = (x_k, y_k)$ in frame I_k and $P_{k+1} = (x_{k+1}, y_{k+1})$ in frame I_{k+1} is a function of the position (x_k, y_k). The chosen scanning broom for the mosaicing process must be a curve $F(x, y) = 0$, perpendicular to the flow vector and close to the centre of the image for minimal lens distortion.

For a horizontal flow, the scanning broom $F(x, y)$ is a vertical straight line, for a vertical flow it is a horizontal straight line and for zoom or forward motion it is a circumference around the center of the known FOE, as shown in Fig. 7 [17].

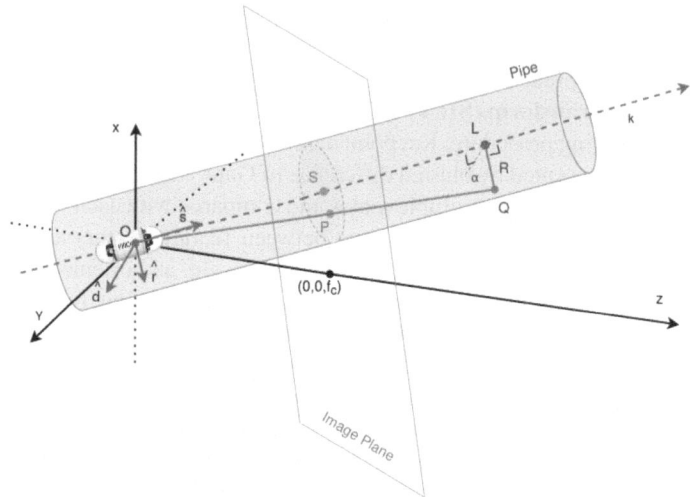

Fig. 5. Diagram illustrating the projection of a 2D planar image (image plane) onto a 3D cylinder (pipe): $s = S/|S|$ is the axis of the pipe; R is the radius; $O = (0,0,0)$ is the optical center; $S = (s_x, s_y, f_c)$ is the focus of expansion; f_c is the focal length and Q is the projection on the pipe of each point $P = (x, y, f_c)$ from the plane [15].

In short, the main steps of the mosaicing process are:

1. the **data association** between image regions that describe the same scene from at least two views. In classical approaches, hand-crafted features are detected, extracted, and matched across the different views. The most explored detectors are Harris, SIFT, SURF, etc., and, more recently, features based on data learned from neural networks. Other methods that do not rely on features are called direct or pixel-based and are formulated as an optimization problem that maximizes a particular similarity metric. More recent strategies resort to the deep learning of regression parameters [11].
2. the **estimation of a geometric transformation** that can robustly map data from different views in a single mosaic.
3. the **smooth blend** of the images for the mosaic.

1.3 Homography Matrix Estimation

Projective geometry studies the properties of a projective plane $\mathbb{IP}^2$ given a set of invertible linear transformations of homogeneous coordinates that map lines to lines. A mapping is a projectivity if and only if there exists a non-singular 3×3 matrix H such that for any point in $\mathbb{IP}^2$ represented by a vector x it is true that $h(x) = Hx$, where H is the homography matrix. From the nine elements of H, only eight ratios are independent, so this transformation has eight degrees of freedom, and collinearity is preserved under the mapping [7]. H can traditionally be obtained from a set of correspondences between two images, using Singular Value Decomposition (SVD) and the Random Sample Consensus (RANSAC) algorithm for outlier removal [15]. In [25], an unsupervised deep homography estimation method with a novel architectural design is introduced. It is inspired by the RANSAC procedure in traditional methods. The learning of an outlier mask is able to selectively identify reliable regions for homography estimation. Instead of directly comparing image content as done in prior methods, the a customized triplet loss is formulated for the network is calculated with respect to the learned deep features.

1.4 Image Quality Assessment

Evaluating the integrity of the result of a mosaicing process with low quality medical and its quality to human perception is a challenge. No-Reference (NR) or blind Image Quality Assessment (IQA) algorithms are used to estimate the quality of a degraded or newly generated image given no ground truth reference image or even the type of processing the image is subjected to. These are commonly used for the quality assessment of compressed images. A few CNN-based NR-IQA models have already been developed in the past years, such as CNNIQA [12], CONTRastive Image QUality Evaluator (CONTRIQUE) [9], and VIDGIQA [6]. For all three above-mentioned models, the higher the value, the higher the quality of the image.

Outline

In the *Related Work* section, we examine previous attempts of panorama construction using a forward-motion camera inside a tubular structure. In the *Dataset* section, our initial dataset of multi-camera WCE videos is discussed and an explanation for the creation of a synthetic model is offered. In the *Methodology* section, we present the principles that our procedure was based on, describe the specific steps taken to build a local forward or backward-motion panorama and the evaluation metrics used to assess the result. In the *Results and Discussion* section, the output of each step of the methodology is presented and some possible alternative paths are addressed. Finally, in the *Conclusion* section, we provide a brief overview of the work developed and discuss the steps of the future work.

2 Related Work

Previous methods for generating panorama images of tubular-shaped organs use 2D images from the oesophagus and a tubular model such as cylindrical projection. The frames are unwrapped around a previously computed centre of projection and mapped into a cylindrical surface based on the camera motion estimation between sequential frames [10, 18].

Behrens et al. developed an image mosaicing algorithm for local panorama construction from bladder video sequences in fluorescence conventional endoscopy. The frames were transformed using an affine parameter model with iterative optimization and stitched together to construct a panoramic image. Some visual artefacts inevitably produced by non-homogeneous lighting were compensated in the stitching step with a mutual linear interpolation function [1]. *Spyrou et al.* proposed an approach that automatically assembled a visual summary using WCE videos based on pipe projection. The frames were geometrically transformed with feature matching techniques and stitched together, providing a broader field of view without information loss [20].

Cao et al. proposed an approach for the generation of an unfolded image of a borehole from Axial View Panoramic Borehole Televiewer (APBT) videos. The sequence of images were unfolded with Daugman's rubber sheet model (RSM) and then fused with an interpolation algorithm to generate a panorama with a projection registration algorithm. The feature extraction process is challenging due to poor image quality and the probe's slight rotation along the central axis of the borehole. This approach is valuable to consider given the similarity in the geometry of the problem [3].

K. Yoshimoto et al. developed a prototype stereo endoscopy with a compound eye system named Thin Observation Module by Bound Optics (TOMBO) for depth mapping from 2D frames to 3D data. They later proposed a procedure for acquiring 3D panoramas of the oesophagus from conventional endoscopy. The methodology involved acquiring a set of frames with an endoscope, reconstructing the corresponding 3D surfaces and estimating its position using scene flow and surface merging. This approach improved the quality of the images by lowering missing points from low-resolution and stereo-matching failures. Validation was performed with a phantom and a pig oesophagus for the size of the texture and the moving distance [24].

3 Dataset

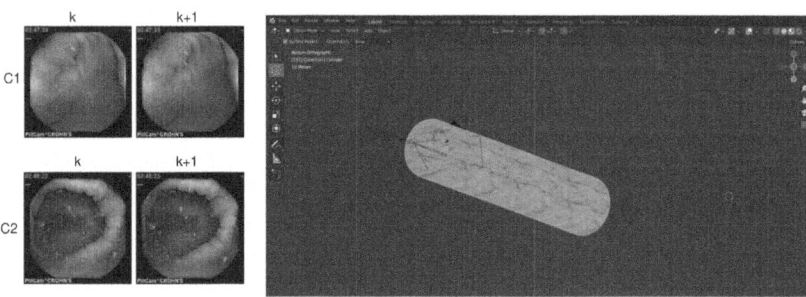

Fig. 6. (Left) Example sample of sequential frames (k and k+1) from a patient's exam video, obtained with the front and back camera (C1 and C2) of a PillCam Colon2 capsule; (Right) Tubular model, created with the Blender Software, with colon-like textured walls, two opposing cameras coupled with light sources animated along a pure translation trajectory [15].

The goal is to obtain the local panoramic views from the consecutive frames of WCE videos from patients with Crohn's disease obtained specifically from the multi-camera capsule PillCam Colon2. At this stage, a synthetic dataset for an initial proof of concept was constructed in order to provide ground truth information regarding motion. For this reason, a colon-like texture tubular model was created with the Blender Software given a few restrictions.

The model, as shown in Fig. 6 (Right), consisted of a hollow tubular structure created with the projection of a colon-like texture. Two cameras were coupled, placed facing opposing directions and added at one end of the tube and animated to follow the pre-defined path. The animation of the purely translational displacement of each camera was rendered with lighting condition variations as the result of a light source that accompanies the motion of each camera. This synthetic model allowed for the division of the entire procedure of building a panorama into smaller steps.

4 Methodology

Unlike conventional endoscopic or geological exploration probes, the capsule used in WCE moves in a translational, resulting in radial pixel displacement in consecutive frames during forward motion and backward motion, with flow vectors pointing outwards during forward motion and inwards during backward motion, as seen in Fig. 4a). When the capsule undergoes pure rotation around its optical axis, the displacement of pixels from sequential frames can be described as clockwise/counterclockwise motion, as shown in Fig. 4b).

Since the movement of the capsule inside the colon is the result of the peristaltic movements of the tissue, its displacement is composed of periods rotation and translation. We will first address the problem assuming no composed motion, only pure rotation or pure translation. Since the sequential frames associated with pure rotation do not offer additional pixels for the panorama, we are only interested in successive frames from pure translation motion periods.

Our approach for handling forward motion and zoom in panorama construction is based on the generalized pipe representation proposed by *Rousso et al.* with a few constraints and adaptations given the specificity of our dataset, as shown in Fig. 5 [17].

Coordinate System Transformation. Since straight optical flow is easier to operate, to simplify the mosaicing process, the set of sequential frames were converted from cartesian coordinates to polar coordinates, as shown in Fig. 8, using Eq. (2) [15], with radius r and angular coordinate θ.

$$\begin{cases} x = rcos(\theta) \\ y = rsin(\theta) \end{cases} \quad (2)$$

Additionally, a bilinear interpolation algorithm was used to interpolate between points that do not lay in the image. Each channel of each RGB frame was converted from cartesian to polar coordinates and then all channels were coupled to obtain each RGB polar frame (Fig. 9).

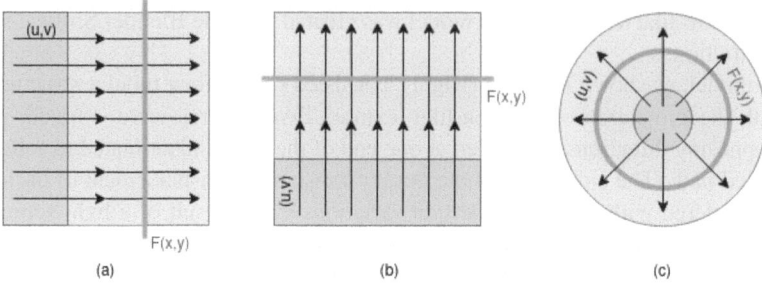

Fig. 7. Given OF as a function of the position, the scanning broom $F(x, y) = 0$ chosen for the mosaicing process must be perpendicular to (u,v): (a) $F(x, y)$ is a vertical straight line for uniform horizontal OF; (b) $F(x, y)$ is a horizontal straight line for uniform vertical OF; (c) $F(x, y)$ is a circumference centred around the FOE for radial OF [15].

4.1 Image Registration

In this methodology, the RAFT network [22] is used to compute flow vectors for the optical flow-based registration. Optical flow measures per-pixel motion estimation between video frames, and a dense displacement field maps each pixel in one frame to the corresponding coordinates in another. The RAFT network consists of a feature encoder, a correlation layer, and a recurrent update operator, which selects values from correlation volumes and updates the flow field. With deep learning, features and motion priors are learned instead of handcrafted. However, the design of architectures with faster and easier training procedures, better performances, and adequate generalization capabilities is still a necessity [22].

Pairwise point correspondences between frames can be established by the flow field [11]. From each pair of consecutive polar frames, the corresponding subset of P^i_{k+1} points coordinates in frame $k + 1$ were computed using a linear interpolation algorithm given the subset of points P^i_k associated with each pixel i from frame k and the optical flow (u^i_k, v^i_k) obtained with the RAFT Network.

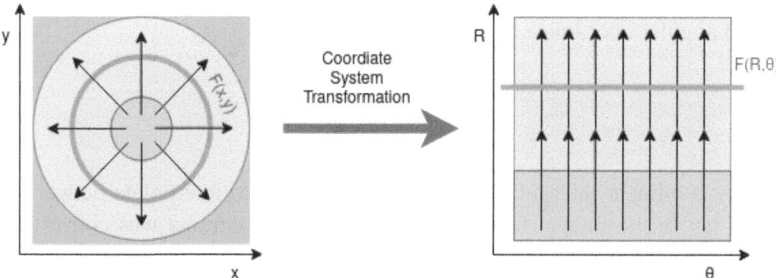

Fig. 8. Coordinate system conversion from cartesian to polar image coordinates (with a central FOE) in order to obtain frames with a straight optical flow pattern and apply a straight scanning broom in the mosaicing process. [15]

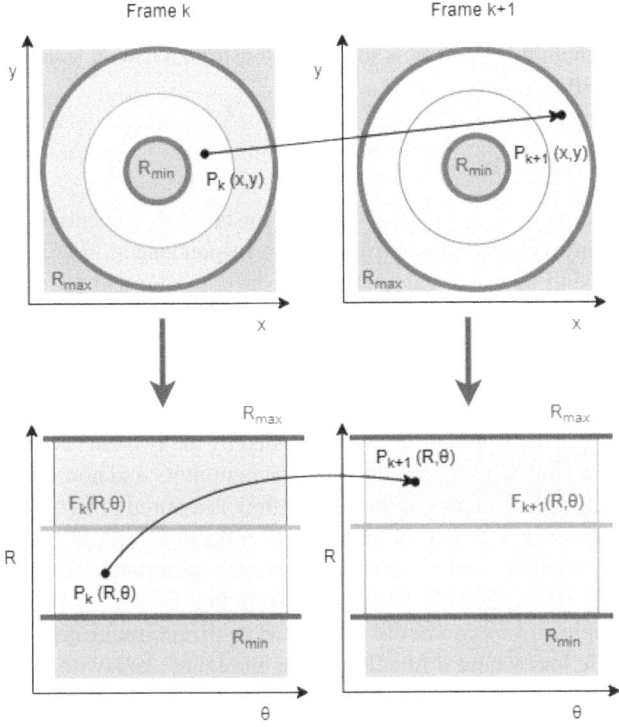

Fig. 9. Diagram illustration of the difference between a point correspondence between two sequential cartesian frames and the corresponding two sequential polar frames after the coordinate system conversion (with a central FOE) [15].

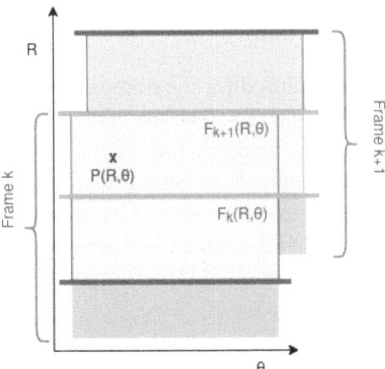

Fig. 10. Ideal mosaicing result given a perfect overlay between the two corresponding points in both frame k and k+1 [15].

This point correspondence is performed for the final panorama mosaicing, and the homography estimation procedure is identical to estimation with sparse feature correspondences like SIFT features.

4.2 Homography Matrix

In this methodology, for each pair of purely translational sequential polar frames, a global homography H is obtained from the correspondences (P_k, P_{k+1}), such that $P_{k+1} = HP_k$, using Singular Value Decomposition (SVD) and the Random Sample Consensus (RANSAC) algorithm for outlier removal. The final mosaic is obtained by warping the set of strips retrieved from the sequential images given the point correspondences. Each strip must be warped to match the boundaries of the previous stitched strips [17].

In our case, from the frame k, the strip bounded by the two curves $F_k(r, \theta) = 0$ and $F'_{k+1}(r, \theta) = 0$, as shown in Fig. 10, ensuring the continuity and non-redundancy of the information, as the orthogonality of the optical flow is assured [17].

The strip bounded by the two curves $F_k(r, \theta) = 0$ and $F'_{k+1}(r, \theta) = 0$ from frame k is used to ensure continuity and non-redundancy of the information, as the orthogonality of the optical flow is assured [17], such as shown in Fig. 10.

The homography matrix can be also estimated by **direct image registration (DRG) with photometric loss** where a function warps the image k+1 with transformation **T** [11]. By transforming the image k+1 into a new position it is possible to obtain k+1 in its new position. The intensity difference of frames k and k+1 can be computed with the L2 norm and the the optimal transformation can be obtained by minimising the loss.

$$H^{drg}_{i,j+1} = arg\ min_{H_{i,j+1}} ||I_k - \mathbf{T}(I_{k+1}, H_{i,j+1})|| \tag{3}$$

The optimisation of Eq. 3 [11, 15] is based the minimization of the least-square difference between a fixed imageframe k and a warped moving image k+1 and the optimisation is solved with the Levenberg-Marquardt iterative algorithm.

4.3 Image Registration Evaluation

To compare the three methods explored for the homography estimation, the inlier ratio was obtained as one of the first metrics. The absolute distances between each transformed point $P'_{k+1} = HP_k$ and its correspondence in the transformed image P_{k+1} were also obtained given each homography H to get a transform-forward (TF) distance and its transpose H^T to get a transform-backwards (TB) distance. The distances explored were the Euclidean, Minkowski (Mink), which is a generalization of the Euclidean and Manhattan distance metrics, and Hamming (Ham) distances. For an ideal registration, these distances would be equal to zero.

For the better performing registration method, additional metrics were obtained. The accuracy of the registration method can be evaluated by the intensity difference of the registered image pair using the Sum of Squared Differences (SSD), which is sensitive to smaller samples with large intensity differences. SSD can be computed over the region R for a transformation $h_{k,k-1}$ that maps a point in image I_k to point x in I_{k-1}, where

R = [x1, x2, ···, xN] is a subset of points in I_{k-1} [15]. For an ideal set of registrations, SSD will equal zero [19].

$$SSD_{k,R} = \sum_{x=x_1}^{x_N} (I_k(h_{k,k-1}(x)) - I_{k-1}(x))^2 \qquad (4)$$

When a registration method performs well, the registered image is as close as possible to the target image, and its average intensity image is the sharpest [19]. The sharpness of the average intensity image is measured by computing the intensity variance of the registered images. Given a transformation $h_{k,k-1}$ that maps a point in image I_k to point x in I_{k-1}, where R is a subset of points in I_{k-1}, the Intensity Variance (IV) of image I_k registered to image I_{k-1}, over the region R, is computed as expressed in Eqs. 5 and 6 [15]. For an ideal registration, IV will be equal to zero.

$$IV_{k,R}(x) = \sum_{x=x_1}^{x_N} (I_{k-1}(h_{k-1,i}(x)) - ave_k(x))^2 \qquad (5)$$

$$ave_k(x) = \frac{1}{N} \sum_{x=x_1}^{x_N} I_k(h_{k-1,k}(x)) \qquad (6)$$

The correlation coefficient measures the linear dependence between two registered images, assuming their intensity relationship is linear. With a transformation $h_{k,k-1}$ that maps a point in image I_k to point x in I_{k-1}, where R is a subset of points in I_{k-1}, the CC of an image I_k registered to image I_{k-1}, over the region R, can be computed, as shown in Eqs. 7, 8, 9 [15]. The ideal CC, given a pair of perfectly registered images, is equal to one [19].

$$d_{k-1}(x) = I_{k-1}(h_{k-1,k}(x)) - \overline{I_{k-1}} \qquad (7)$$

$$d_k(x) = I_k(x) - \overline{I_k} \qquad (8)$$

$$CC_{i,R} = \frac{\sum_{x=x_1}^{x_N} d_{k-1}(x) d_k(x)}{\sqrt{\sum_{x=x_1}^{x_N} d_{k-1}(x)^2 \sum_{x=x_1}^{x_N} d_k(x)^2}} \qquad (9)$$

4.4 Image Quality Assessment

In order to have a quantitative evaluation of our final local forward and backward-motion, central and non-central, panoramas obtained after the polar image stitching process, the NR-IQA models CNNIQA [12], CONTRastive Image QUality Evaluator (CONTRIQUE) [9] and VIDGIQA [6] m previously mentioned were used, their values were computed and compared with the results from a pre-trained Unsupervised Deep Homography (UDH) network [25] given our image sequences.

4.5 Motion Segmentation of Multi-camera WCE Videos

Assuming that rotation and translation do not occur simultaneously, the multi-camera PillCam Colon2 dataset allows for the extraction of frames that correspond to pure translation motion by analyzing the pixel displacement between sequential frames from both cameras at the same instant. The optical flow between sequential frames from both cameras of the same capsule were manually chosen from the flow field distribution obtained with the RAFT network [22]. The frames were converted into polar coordinates and vertical flow fields were extracted so that pure translational motion segments were chosen.

5 Results and Discussion

Figure 11 shows a sample pair of consecutive synthetic frames obtained from the video rendered from the Blender model and each corresponding polar representation after the coordinate system conversion, presented in Eq. 2, assuming a central FOE. Figure 12 shows another pair of two consecutive frames from another video rendered from the Blender model with a non-central but known FOE. A methodology needs to be developed for the computation of the FOE in cases that are non-central to apply this pipeline to a real-case scenario with the multi-camera capsule images.

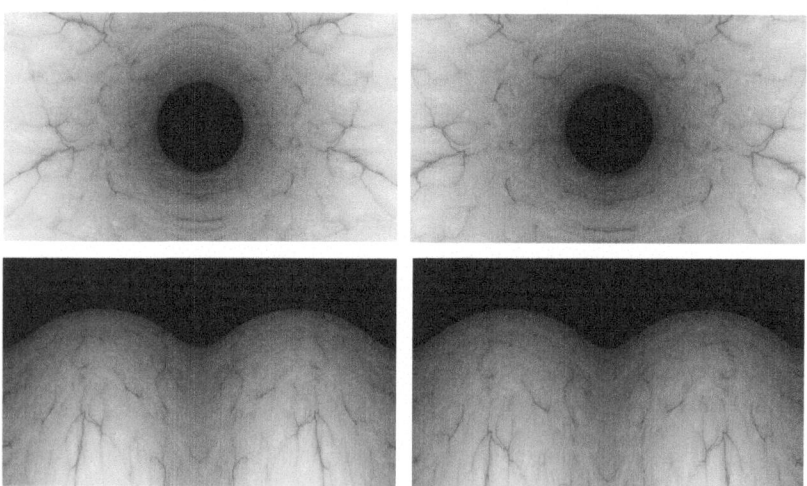

Fig. 11. Sample example of two consecutive frames rendered from the colon-like synthetic blender model and the corresponding two sequential polar frames after the coordinate system conversion with a central FOE.

Figure 13 compares the ratio of inliers between each of the three methods explored for homography computation for 15 consecutive pairs of frames. The optical flow results and direct registration results are similar since both offer consistently lower

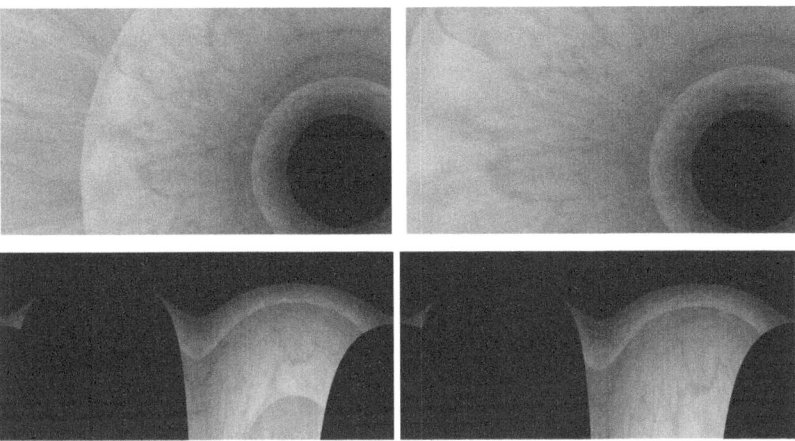

Fig. 12. Sample example of two consecutive frames rendered from the colon-like synthetic blender model and the corresponding two sequential polar frames after the coordinate system conversion with a non-central FOE.

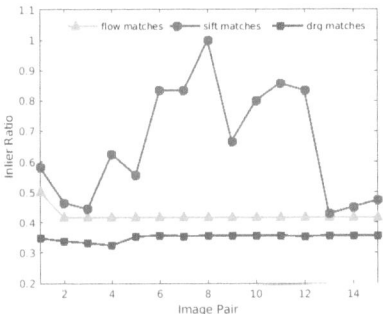

Fig. 13. Inlier Ratio using Optical Flow Point Correspondences, SIFT matches or Direct Registration from a forward-motion image sequence of 15 image pairs.

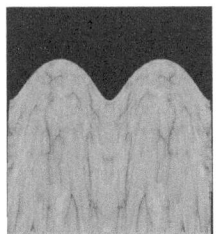 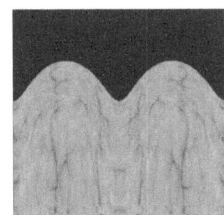 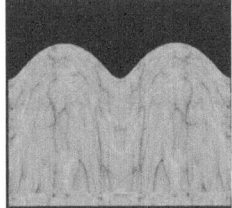

Fig. 14. Mosaicing result with Direct Registration (left), Optical Flow Point Correspondences (middle) and SIFT matches (right).

inlier ratios. SIFT offers a small number of correspondence despite having a higher inlier ratio. Figure 14 shows the final panorama mosaic for each of the three methods. Visually, the worst result is obtained with SIFT since the mosaic looks stretched. The best visual results are obtained with the optical flow correspondences since it offers a better seam between successive frames. Figure 15 shows the inlier ratios for different down-sampling ratios of the original sample. It shows how the sample size influences the inlier ratio. There seems to be an optimal value of down-sample ratio that allows for better inlier ratio values. The upcoming results were obtained with the optical flow method with the optimal down-sample ratio.

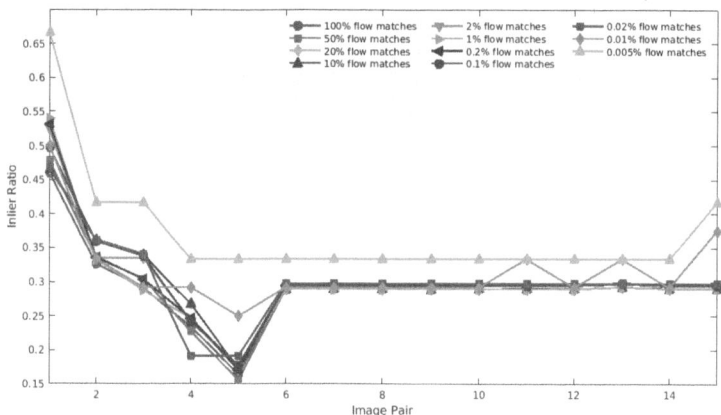

Fig. 15. Inlier Ratio using Optical Flow point correspondences (flow matches) with different sample sizes from a forward-motion image sequence of 15 image pairs.

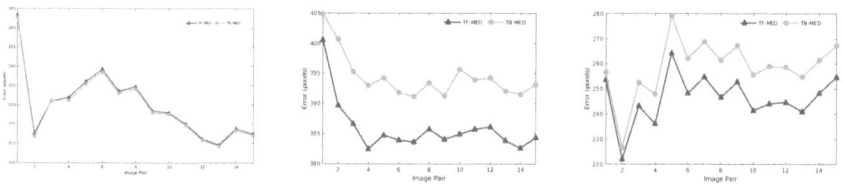

Fig. 16. Transform-Forward and Transform-Backward Mean Euclidean Distance (TF-MED and TB-MED) for Direct Registration (Left), SIFT matches (middle) and Optical Flow Correspondences (right).

Figure 16 presents the Transform-Forward and Transform-Backward Mean Euclidean Distance (TF-MED and TB-MED) between each pair of frames for the corresponding homography estimated with the direct registration method, the sift algorithm and the optical flow correspondences. Figure 17 shows the TF and TB values for the mean Minkowski and the mean Hamming distance for all three methods.

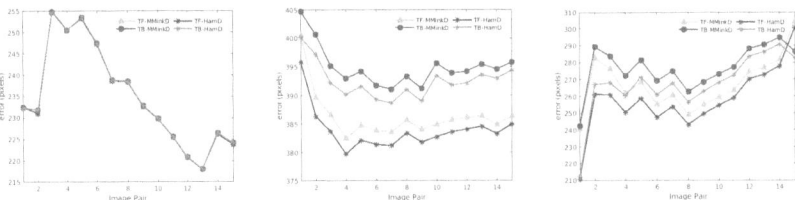

Fig. 17. Transform-Forward and Transform-Backward Mean Minkowski Distance (TF-MMinkD and TB-MMinkD) and Transform-Forward and Transform-Backward Hamming Distance (TF-MHamD and TB-MHamD) for Direct Registration (left), SIFT matches (middle) and Optical Flow Correspondences (right).

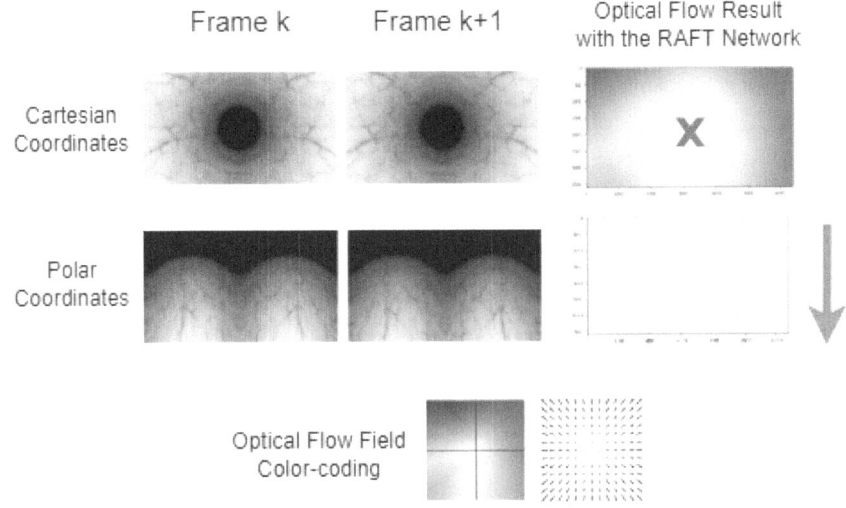

Fig. 18. Sample example of two consecutive frames rendered from the colon-like synthetic blender model, the corresponding two sequential polar frames after the coordinate system conversion with a central FOE and the associated Optical Flow field result for each case.

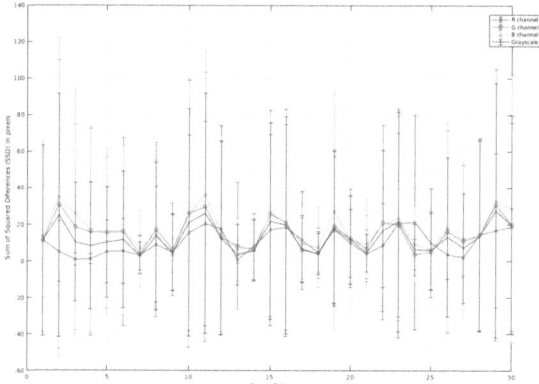

Fig. 19. SSD between each image I_{k+1} and its previous one I_k for the intensities of each RGB channel and for grayscale, for all 30 pairs of consecutive frames from the video rendered with the Blender Software.

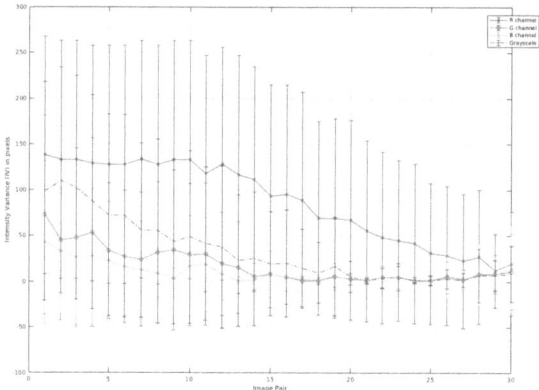

Fig. 20. IV between each image I_{k+1} and its previous one I_k for the intensities of each RGB channel and for grayscale, for all 30 pairs of consecutive frames from the video rendered with the Blender Software.

Figure 18 shows the optical flow result obtained with the RAFT network given the polar representation of the consecutive frames. The output color of this example is all yellow, corresponding to the vertical flow field as expected since the displacement of the capsule is designed to be purely translational in our Blender model. Figures 19, 20, 21 show the values of the metrics SSD, IV, and CC between each image I_{k+1} and the previous one I_k, given the homography computed from the optical flow matches, for each one of the intensities of each RGB channel and its grayscale, for all 30 pairs of consecutive frames assessed from the rendered video.

Figure 22 shows the final panorama obtained after the mosaicing process of the full 30 pairs of consecutive frames from the forward-motion video with the blender model.

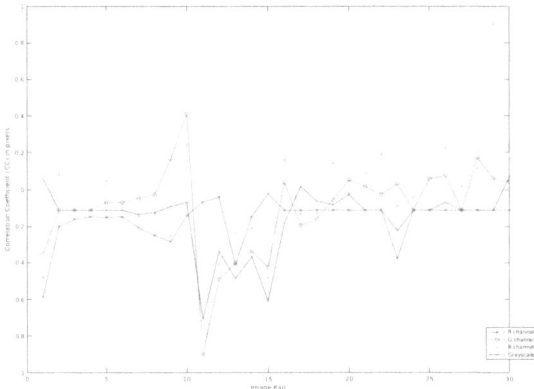

Fig. 21. CC between each image I_{k+1} and its previous one I_k for the intensities of each RGB channel and for grayscale, for all 30 pairs of consecutive frames from the video rendered with the Blender Software.

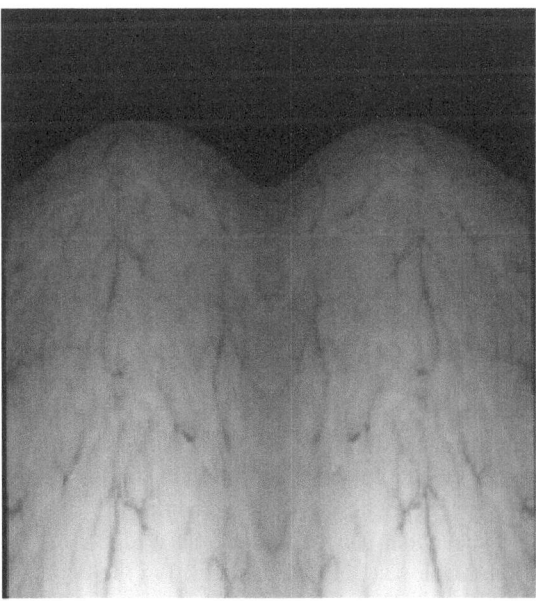

Fig. 22. Example of a final panorama, in this case, a local and central FOE forward-motion panorama obtained from the mosaicing of all 30 pairs of consecutive polar frames given one video rendered from the tubular Blender model.

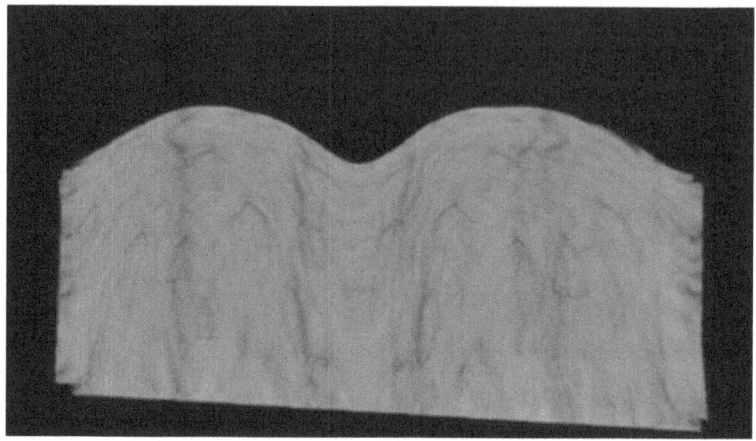

Fig. 23. Example of a local, in this case forward-motion with central FOE, of the panorama result with an Unsupervised Deep Homography (UDH) network [13].

Table 1. Blind or No-reference Image Quality Assessment (NR-IQA): CNNIQA [12], CONTRIQUE [9] and VIDGIQA [6] normalized values ([0,1]) of the local forward-motion (FM) and backward-motion (BM) panoramas with central FOE (C-FOE) and with non-central FOE (NC-FOE), obtained with the traditional approach for a global homography estimation (GH) using the RANSAC algorithm with the optical flow derived correspondences estimated with the RAFT network and with an Unsupervised Deep Homography (UDH) network [14].

Dataset		CNNIQA		CONTRIQUE		VIDGIQA	
		GH	UDH	GH	UDH	GH	UDH
FM	C-FOE	0.267	**0.274**	0.478	**0.432**	0.114	**0.309**
	NC-FOE	0.270	**0.545**	0.196	**0.326**	0.511	**0.795**
BM	C-FOE	0.329	**0.370**	0.289	**0.259**	0.190	**0.490**
	NC-FOE	0.346	**0.463**	0.151	**0.249**	0.527	**0.555**

Figure 23 shows the final mosaic of a panoramic view obtained with a state of the art Unsupervised Deep Homography (UDH) network [14]. Table 1 shows the normalized NR-IQA values for the final local panorama from Fig. 22 obtained with our global homography (GH) methodology given the three above-mentioned CNN-based IQA models and its comparison with the UDIS network.

Figure 24 shows a sequential pair of frames retrieved from a WCE video from a patient with the PillCam Colon2. Both frames are from the two cameras on opposite sides of the capsule (C1 and C2), in cartesian and polar coordinates, and the corresponding optical flow estimation from the polar representation with the RAFT network.

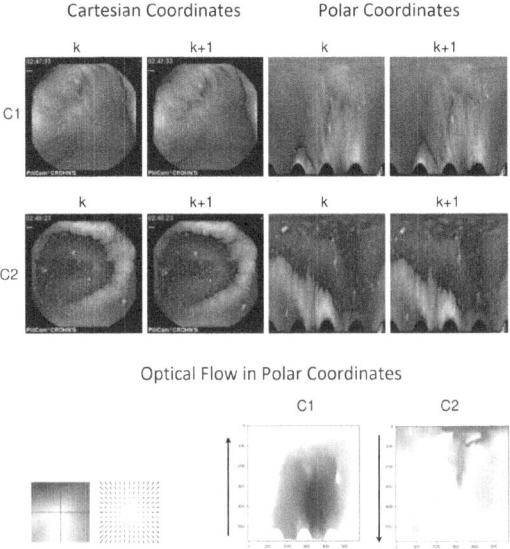

Fig. 24. Example of a sequential pair of frames from the cameras on both ends of the capsule (C1 and C2) and the optical flow estimation given the polar representation with the RAFT network [22].

6   Conclusions and Future Work

The registration results are satisfactory, but the IQA results from the final panorama are far from ideal. Further exploration of a more robust methodology for the mosaicing process is needed, such as computing several local homographies instead of a global one, exploring non-classical deep learning tools for iterative stitching or fusing more than one approach. Further research work is also required to deal with the discontinuities where the boundaries of each strip are visible, creating artefacts that lower the image quality.

Additionally, a robust metric for a quantitative comparison of the OF vector field of consecutive frames from the opposing end cameras (C1 and C2) is also needed to use as a segmentation criterion for a non-manual motion segmentation process.

The UDH neural network presents better results with the IQA models explored, but visually it is possible to perceive that the final result is degraded, the quality of the final images is inferior, the overlay of the images is worse, and the content of the image becomes less perceptible and distinguishable. We can conclude that the approach explored is more adequate for the intended purpose. A more realistic synthetic dataset with more variability would allow for further exploration of the potential of this approach.

The future goal is the computation of these local panoramas with the patient videos, given that the purely translational frames correspond to backward and forward motion from both back and front cameras, which are rigidly connected and that both correspond essentially to a vertical OF vector field in polar coordinates, as shown in Fig. 24.

Acknowledgment. The authors would like to acknowledge the support of project PTDC/EMD-EMD/28960/2017, entitled "Multi-Cam Capsule Endoscopy Imagery: 3D Capsule Location and Detection of Abnormalities", funded by FCT, the PhD Scholarship 2020.06592.BD funded by FCT, and the Institute of Systems and Robotics - University of Coimbra, under project the with DOI 10.54499/UIDB/00048/2020, funded by FCT.

References

1. Behrens, A.: Creating panoramic images for bladder fluorescence endoscopy. Acta Polytechnica **48** (2008). https://doi.org/10.14311/1013
2. Brown, A.P., Jayatissa, A.H.: Analysis of current and future technologies of capsule endoscopy: a mini review. Arch. Prev. Med. **5**(1), 031–034 (2020)
3. Cao, M., Deng, Z., Rai, L., Teng, S., Zhao, M., Collier, M.: Generating panoramic unfolded image from borehole video acquired through APBT. Multimedia Tools Appl. **77**(19), 25149–25179 (2018). https://doi.org/10.1007/s11042-018-5779-x
4. Ciuti, G., Menciassi, A., Dario, P.: Capsule endoscopy: from current achievements to open challenges. IEEE Rev. Biomed. Eng. **4**, 59–72 (2011)
5. Figueiredo, I.N., Pinto, L., Perdigoto, L., Oliveira, M., Araújo, H., Figueiredo, P.N.: Wireless capsule endoscope location and a robotic validation experiment, pp. 1361–1365 (2019)
6. Guan, J., Yi, S., Zeng, X., Cham, W.K., Wang, X.: Visual importance and distortion guided deep image quality assessment framework. IEEE Trans. Multimedia **19**(11), 2505–2520 (2017). https://doi.org/10.1109/TMM.2017.2703148
7. Hartley, R., Zisserman, A.: Multiple View Geometry in Computer Vision. Cambridge University Press, Cambridge (2003). https://books.google.pt/books?id=eLbfoQEACAAJ
8. Iakovidis, D., Tsevas, S., Polydorou, A.: Reduction of capsule endoscopy reading times by unsupervised image mining. Comput. Med. Imaging Graph. **34**(6), 471–478 (2010). https://doi.org/10.1016/j.compmedimag.2009.11.005. https://www.sciencedirect.com/science/article/pii/S0895611109001372. Biomedical Image Technologies and Methods - BIBE 2008
9. Kang, L., Ye, P., Li, Y., Doermann, D.: Convolutional neural networks for no-reference image quality assessment. In: Proceedings of the IEEE Computer Society Conference on Computer Vision and Pattern Recognition, pp. 1733–1740 (2014). https://doi.org/10.1109/CVPR.2014.224
10. Kim, R., et al.: Quantitative endoscopy: precise computerized measurement of metaplastic epithelial surface area in barrett's esophagus. Gastroenterology **108**(2), 360–366 (1995). https://doi.org/10.1016/0016-5085(95)90061-6. https://www.sciencedirect.com/science/article/pii/0016508595900616
11. Li, L., et al.: Robust endoscopic image mosaicking via fusion of multimodal estimation. Med. Image Anal. **84**, 102709 (2023). https://doi.org/10.1016/j.media.2022.102709
12. Madhusudana, P.C., Birkbeck, N., Wang, Y., Adsumilli, B., Bovik, A.C.: Image quality assessment using contrastive learning. IEEE Trans. Image Process. **31**, 4149–4161 (2022). https://doi.org/10.1109/tip.2022.3181496
13. Nguyen, T., Chen, S.W., Shivakumar, S.S., Taylor, C.J., Kumar, V.: Unsupervised deep homography: a fast and robust homography estimation model. IEEE Robot. Autom. Lett. **3**(3) (2018)
14. Nie, L., Lin, C., Liao, K., Liu, S., Zhao, Y.: Unsupervised deep image stitching: reconstructing stitched features to images. IEEE Trans. Image Process. **30**, 6184–6197 (2021). https://doi.org/10.1109/TIP.2021.3092828

15. Oliveira, M., Araujo, H.: Local forward-motion panoramic views for localization and lesion detection for multi-camera wireless capsule endoscopy videos. In: Proceedings of the 16th International Joint Conference on Biomedical Engineering Systems and Technologies (BIOSTEC 2023) - Volume 3: BIOINFORMATICS, pp. 41–50. INSTICC, SciTePress (2023). https://doi.org/10.5220/0011626600003414
16. Oliveira, M., Araujo, H., Figueiredo, I.N., Pinto, L., Curto, E., Perdigoto, L.: Registration of consecutive frames from wireless capsule endoscopy for 3D motion estimation. IEEE Access **9**, 119533–119545 (2021). https://doi.org/10.1109/ACCESS.2021.3108234
17. Rousso, B., Peleg, S., Finci, I., Rav-Acha, A.: Universal mosaicing using pipe projection. In: Proceedings of the IEEE International Conference on Computer Vision, pp. 945–952 (1998). https://doi.org/10.1109/iccv.1998.710830
18. Seibel, E.J., et al.: Tethered capsule endoscopy, a low-cost and high-performance alternative technology for the screening of esophageal cancer and Barrett's esophagus. IEEE Trans. Biomed. Eng. **55**(3), 1032–1042 (2008). https://doi.org/10.1109/TBME.2008.915680
19. Song, J.H.: Methods for evaluating image registration. The University of Iowa (2017)
20. Spyrou, E., Diamantis, D., Iakovidis, D.K.: Panoramic visual summaries for efficient reading of capsule endoscopy videos, pp. 41–46 (2013). https://doi.org/10.1109/SMAP.2013.21
21. Swain, P.: Wireless capsule endoscopy. Gut **52**(suppl 4), iv48–iv50 (2003). https://doi.org/10.1136/gut.52.suppl_4.iv48. https://gut.bmj.com/content/52/suppl_4/iv48
22. Teed, Z., Deng, J.: RAFT: recurrent all-pairs field transforms for optical flow (extended abstract). In: IJCAI International Joint Conference on Artificial Intelligence, pp. 4839–4843 (2021). https://doi.org/10.24963/ijcai.2021/662
23. Třebický, V., Fialová, J., Kleisner, K., Havlíček, J.: Focal length affects depicted shape and perception of facial images. PLoS ONE **11**(2), 1–14 (2016). https://doi.org/10.1371/journal.pone.0149313
24. Yoshimoto, K., et al.: Three-dimensional panorama image of tubular structure using stereo endoscopy. Int. J. Innovative Comput. Inf. Control **16**(3) (2020)
25. Zhang, J., et al.: Content-aware unsupervised deep homography estimation. In: Vedaldi, A., Bischof, H., Brox, T., Frahm, J.-M. (eds.) ECCV 2020. LNCS, vol. 12346, pp. 653–669. Springer, Cham (2020). https://doi.org/10.1007/978-3-030-58452-8_38

Estimation of Fluid Intake Volume from Surface Electromyography Signals: A Comparative Study Between Subject-Specific and Global Regression Techniques

Iman A. Ismail[✉] and Ernest N. Kamavuako

Department of Engineering, King's College London, London, UK
{iman.a.ismail,ernest.kamavuako}@kcl.ac.uk
https://www.kcl.ac.uk

Abstract. Insufficient fluid intake in older adults is a prevalent and concerning health issue with far-reaching implications. Monitoring fluid intake is particularly important in various healthcare settings, including hospitals, long-term care facilities, and home care, as well as for specific populations such as older adults or individuals with certain medical conditions. This paper presents an investigation to estimate the fluid intake volume using surface Electromyographic (sEMG) sensors. Eleven subjects participated in the experiment, and sEMG recordings of swallows from cups, bottles, and straws were collected. Four features were extracted from the EMG signals. Seven regression algorithms were implemented for quantifying the volume of swallowed fluid: Random Forest (RF), Support Vector Regressor, K-nearest neighbour (KNN), Linear Regressor (LR), Decision Tree (DT), Lasso, and Ridge. The mean sip volume across subjects was 14.85 ± 5.05 ml. Results showed that using Random Forest as a subject-specific regressor, the root mean square (RMSE) for estimating fluid intake volume using the Mean Absolute Value feature gave 1.37 ± 1.1 ml, and using Support Vector as a global regressor, the RMSE was 2.5 ± 1.2 ml using the Waveform Length feature. When applied as global regressors, SVR gave 6.04 ± 1.7 ml with the Mel Frequency Cepstrum Coefficients feature and 6.36 ± 1.6 ml with the Willison Amplitude feature. Random Forest gave 6.04 ± 1.7 ml with the Willison Amplitude feature. These results indicate a step forward in estimating fluid intake volume based on sEMG for hydration monitoring.

Keywords: Dehydration · Electromyography sensors · Fluid intake · Volume quantifying · Swallowing

1 Introduction

Dehydration has significant implications for the health of older adults [1]. Due to reduced thirst sensation for older adults, they may consume less fluid as their bodies become less efficient at maintaining fluid balance [2]. Furthermore, they are more susceptible to conditions that heighten the risk of dehydration, such as kidney disease, diabetes, and certain medications [3]. The ageing process results in older adults having 10 to 15% less water in their bodies, contributing to potential health issues [4]. A comprehensive review indicated that the majority of older adults face heightened vulnerability to renal problems and electrolyte imbalances due to medication-induced dehydration, rendering them more prone to fluctuations in health conditions and illnesses [4].

Fluid charts represent a vital clinical tool in hospitals and care facilities, allowing nurses to monitor patients' fluid intake and output over the day [5]. Despite their importance, fluid charts have limitations, as nurses may occasionally overlook recording a patient's intake [6]. As Asogan (2021) mentioned, only 25% of fluid charts at Kettering General Hospital contained precise measurements, and only 14% provided comprehensive records of all intakes and outputs [7]. This underscores the necessity to explore technologies, such as wearable devices, to enhance the precision and monitoring of fluid intake, thereby mitigating the risk of dehydration.

There is a growing interest in the potential of wearable technologies to monitor various aspects of health, including fluid intake [8]. Wearable devices facilitate the capability for real-time monitoring and tracking of fluid consumption. Several wearable technologies, such as accelerometers, inertial sensors, smartwatches, cellphones, acoustic sensors, and Electromyography sensors, have been employed to monitor fluid intake [9-14]. These devices are rapidly accessible in the commercial market and have been used to recognize drinking activities, such as drinking from smart containers (cups, bottles, straws, and glasses) and measuring fluid volumes, whether continuous or discrete [6,15]. Nevertheless, their capability to accurately estimate fluid volume remains unreliable, despite research indicating their capability in detecting drinking events using machine learning with an accuracy exceeding 80%.

Furthermore, some older adults dislike these gadgets and prefer not to wear them (Wellnitz, 2019) [16]. For textile techniques to be useful in daily life, they must be connected to the clothing and securely laundered in the washing machine. Respiratory Inductance Plethysmography (RIP), for example, has produced positive results for swallowing detection but hasn't calculated the volume of fluid consumed. Accordingly, none of these methods has been used to quantify the volume of fluid intake in the clinic, despite the encouraging results of these methods for detecting swallowing and drinking events (Dong, 2017; Cheng, 2010 - Tatulli, 2020) [17,18].

While Electromyography (EMG) sensors are primarily known for their application in monitoring and recording the electrical activity produced by muscles, their innovative use in fluid monitoring has emerged as a promising frontier. This novel approach allows for a more comprehensive understanding of how muscular activity influences fluid behaviour, leading to fluid intake detection and volume estimation advancements. The use of physiological sensors to capture swallowing events is based on the fair assumption that fluid consumption can only be confirmed after it has been swallowed. Malvuccio and Kamavuako (2021) employed surface electromyography (sEMG) recordings of individual and continuous swallows to distinguish between liquid and saliva swallows, achieving an accuracy of $86.7 \pm 5.52\%$ through fine K-nearest neighbour(KNN). Furthermore, they attained a classification accuracy of $99.0 \pm 1.30\%$ in distinguishing between noise and swallows using a fine Gaussian support vector machine (SVM) [6]. Additionally, they explored how sEMG features impact the classification of swallowing events and the estimation of fluid volume [19]. Ismail and Kamavuako applied sEMG to estimate fluid intake volume, achieving a root mean square error of 1.37 ± 1.10 mL by applying random forest (RF) with a single feature [20]. Amft and Tröster utilized surface electromyography (EMG) and microphones to continuously monitor swallowing events, aiming to differentiate between solid and liquid meals in a single participant [21].

Vaiman et al. (2003) developed a database using EMG to analyze the duration and amplitude of muscle activities during swallowing and continuous drinking in 100 children. This database serves as a tool for identifying abnormalities in pediatric patients and establishing benchmarks for comparing swallowing performance within and between patients [23]. In a study by Nicholls et al. (2022), EMG was employed to detect eating behaviour coupled with real-time wristband haptic feedback to promote mindful eating. Chewing and swallowing were classified using a support vector machine, yielding F-scores of 0.95 and 0.87, respectively [22]. Nederkoorn et al. (1999) measured swallowing activity through EMG to assess saliva secretion by quantifying peaks in the EMG activity of the musculus digastricus [24]. Vinyard et al. (2016) explored the relationship between food textures and oral processing using EMG, employing it as a general measure of food texture, oral physiology, absolute force, and muscle work [25]. Another innovative study integrated EMG sensors into wearable glasses to measure temporalis muscle activity for detecting intake-related events, achieving 96% accuracy in counting chewing cycles and up to 90.8% accuracy in classifying five types of food [26]. In 2014, Kobayashi et al. used a throat microphone to capture swallowing sounds, achieving a precise fluid intake detection accuracy of 95% through cross-validation of Support Vector Machines (SVM) [27]. Additionally, they estimated the quantity of liquid consumed with a Root Mean Square Error (RMSE) of 3.33 ml, based on the amplitude characteristic of swallowing sound (Kobayashi, 2014).

Although EMG is a promising application in some studies for monitoring food and fluid, the number of studies using sEMG to measure fluid volume is still limited. The challenge is not only to detect and classify liquids but also to estimate the fluid volume. Therefore, this study aims to compare the capability of different regressors in estimating fluid intake volume using sEMG. Novel contributions of this paper include (1) investigating different machine learning regressors to find the optimum regressor in estimating fluid volume (2) unravelling the dependency between the choice of regressor and features, and (3) proposing optimum placement of sEMG electrodes with minimum error (4) comparing between the use of subject-specific and global regression techniques (all subjects pulled together).

2 Methodology

2.1 Dataset

This study uses a previously recorded dataset; details can be found in (Malvuccio Kamavuako, 2021). In brief, three females and eight men, aged 20 to 67 years, participated in this study. Two of the Delsys Tringo sensors were placed on the belly of the suprahyoid muscles, and two were placed on the belly of the infrahyoid muscles. Drinking occurred through various classes (using a cup, straw, bottle, and scale). The recording duration was 10 s for each event. After data checks, two subjects had poor EMG data and were removed from the investigation.

2.2 Experimental Procedure

Subjects consumed water using a bottle, a cup, and a straw, called containers, for simplicity. We used a digital scale to weigh the container before and after drinking to quantify the true sip volume. A sip is a drink, taking only a small amount at a time. For the final group of drinks, 5 ml was added to the highest cup volume that could be computed, and this assignment was only done once.

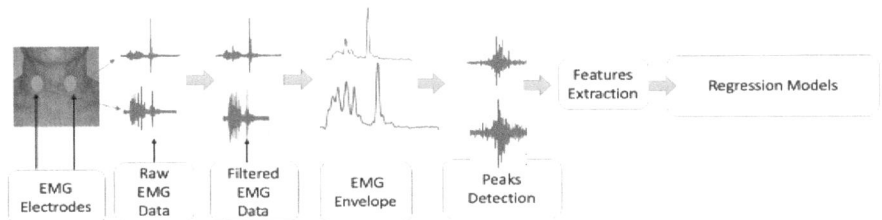

Fig. 1. A graphical representation of the experimental approach and data analysis pipeline [20].

2.3 Data Analysis

On Google Collab, we analysed data using Python 3.8, and preprocessing consisted of bandpass filtering between 6–400 Hz. As shown in Fig. 1, the EMG signals were rectified, and the signal envelope was computed to detect the highest peak where the swallowing event occurred. The EMG burst was then extracted using the peak position. From that burst, features of the Mel frequency cepstral coefficients (MFCCs), Mean Absolute Value (MAV), Waveform Length (WL), and Willison Amplitude (WAMP) were calculated on the raw data of the EMG. These features had positive outcomes when applied to EMG signals in earlier investigations.

– Mean Absolute Value (MAV): It is a method for identifying and evaluating the intensity of muscular contractions. It can be represented as the moving average of the full wave rectified EMG signal, as shown in Eq. 1 [20].

$$MAV = \frac{1}{N} \sum_{i=1}^{N} |X_i| \qquad (1)$$

While N is the length of the segment, i is the segment increment, and Xi is the signal amplitude value.

- Mel-frequency cepstral coefficients (MFCCs): MFCCs are coefficients that form the Mel-frequency cepstrum (MFC) based on a linear cosine transform of a log power spectrum on a nonlinear Mel scale of frequency. It works by segmenting the signal to several windows, then applying the Discrete Fourier Transform (DFT) and taking the log of the magnitude. Then, it wraps the frequencies on a Mel scale and, in the end, applies the inverse Discrete Cosine Transform (DCT).
- Willison Amplitude (WAMP): The WAMP feature counts the number of changes in the amplitude of the EMG signal that surpasses a specific threshold, as shown in Eq. 2 [20].

$$WAMP = \sum_{i=1}^{N}[f(|X_i - X_{i+1}|)]; f(x) = \begin{cases} 1, x >= \text{threshold} \\ 0, \text{otherwise} \end{cases} \quad (2)$$

- Waveform Length (WL): It is the total length of the waveform for the segment. The results obtained from the WL computation indicate the waveform's amplitude, frequency, and duration, as shown in Eq. 3 [20].

$$WL = \sum_{i=1}^{N-1} |X_{i+1} - X_i| \quad (3)$$

We used a regression approach to estimate drinking volume from sEMG. Our analysis included the following techniques: Random Forest (RF), Support Vector Regressor (SVR), K-Nearest Neighbor Regressor (KNN), Linear Regression (LR), Decision Tree (DT), Lasso, and Ridge regressors. Training was implemented as follows: for each subject, we had 16 observations; thus, a leave-one-sample-out was employed with permutation, with the Root Mean Square Error (RMSE) as the performance metric.

In the first part of the data analysis, we investigated the impact of using all four channels versus the two lower (infrahyoid muscles) and upper (suprahyoid muscles) channels using all regressors as subject-specific regressors, single features and all features together. We used a three-way repeated measures analysis of variance (3-ANOVA) with factors (Channels, Regressors and features) to test for statistical differences between the factors and interactions. In the second part of data analysis, we analysed the impact of using all four channels versus the two lower (infrahyoid muscles) and upper (suprahyoid muscles) channels using all regressors as global regressors, single features and all features together. A ten-fold cross-validation technique with normalised features was implemented to get the average RMSE.

In the final part of the data analysis, we selected the three regressors and features with the lowest RMSE to investigate the effect of single and mixed channels (one upper and one lower) on performance. Similarly, we used 3-ANOVA to test for statistical differences. We compared the best three subject-specific and global regressors with the lowest RMSE. We used a two-way repeated measures analysis of variance (2-ANOVA) with factors (Regressors and Features) to test for statistical differences between the factors and interactions. Results are expressed as mean ± standard error.

3 Results

The overall grand mean of the sip volume across subjects and estimation RMSE across channels, regressors, and features were 13.91 ± 1.27 ml and 1.37 ± 0.39 ml using subject-specific regressors and 8.42 ± 1.4 ml using global regressors, respectively.

The Effect of Regressors and Features. Using the subject-specific regressors, the RMSE of all four channels was 2.65 ± 0.32 ml, not significantly lower than the infrahyoid (2.90 ± 0.35 ml) and suprahyoid (2.76 ± 0.33 ml) pairs. There was a statistical difference between regressors (P = 0.003), with RF (2.25 ± 0.25 ml), SVR (2.29 ± 0.30 ml), and KNN (2.41 ± 0.37 ml) performing better than the others, also summarised in Fig. 2. There was no interaction between channels and regressors (P = 0.379).

The mean performance of each feature, in ascending order, was 1.37 ± 0.39 ml for MAV, 1.82 ± 0.45 ml for MFCC, 1.82 ± 0.45 ml for all features combined, 1.99 ± 0.60 ml for WAMP and 2.12 ± 0.44 ml for WL, not statistically different (P = 0.132) from each other. There was an interaction (P = 0.01) between regressors and features, meaning that the choice of features affects the performance of the regressors, as summarised in Table 1. Figure 3 depicts the relationship between regressors and features when using the two suprahyoid muscles. Figure 4 depicts the relationship between regressors and features when using the two infrahyoid muscles, and Fig. 5 depicts the relationship between regressors and features when using the two suprahyoid and the two infrahyoid muscles.

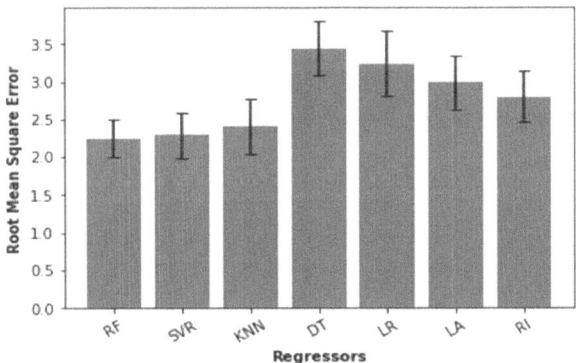

Fig. 2. An error bar plot that summarizes the RMSE and the STD for the seven regressors [20].

Table 1 indicates that performance can be maximised using suprahyoid muscles with Random forest as a subject-specific regressor with the MAV feature. Nevertheless, SVR and KNN are good regressor candidates with the MFCC feature.

Single-channel investigation showed no difference between channels nor their combinations (infrahyoid and suprahyoid). It is worth noting that using the left infrahyoid or left suprahyoid channel alone with the RF regressor with either MAV or MFCC provided RMSE values close to 1.6 ml. The combined left supra and proper infra channels

Table 1. Association between features and best regressor for different channels [20].

Features	Four channels	Infrahyoid muscles	Suprahyoid muscles
MFCC	RF 2.26 ± 0.27 ml	SVR 2.27 ± 0.41 ml	KNN 1.82 ± 0.45 ml
MAV	RF 1.44 ± 0.25 ml	Lasso/Ridge 2.19 ± 0.42 ml	**RF 1.37 ± 0.39 ml**
WAMP	KNN 1.99 ± 0.60 ml	KNN 2.09 ± 0.57 ml	KNN 2.03 ± 0.57 ml
WL	SVR 2.24 ± 0.36 ml	SVR 2.15 ± 0.44 ml	RF 2.12 ± 0.44 ml
ALL	SVR 2.06 ± 0.60 ml	SVR 1.97 ± 0.36 ml	KNN 1.82 ± 0.45 ml

were performed down to 1.5 ml using RF and MAV. The combination of MAV and MFCC using the two suprahyoid channels with the RF has not improved the RMSE results. Table 2 demonstrates the average sip volume and the Root Mean Square error for each subject using the upper two suprahyoid muscles with RF.

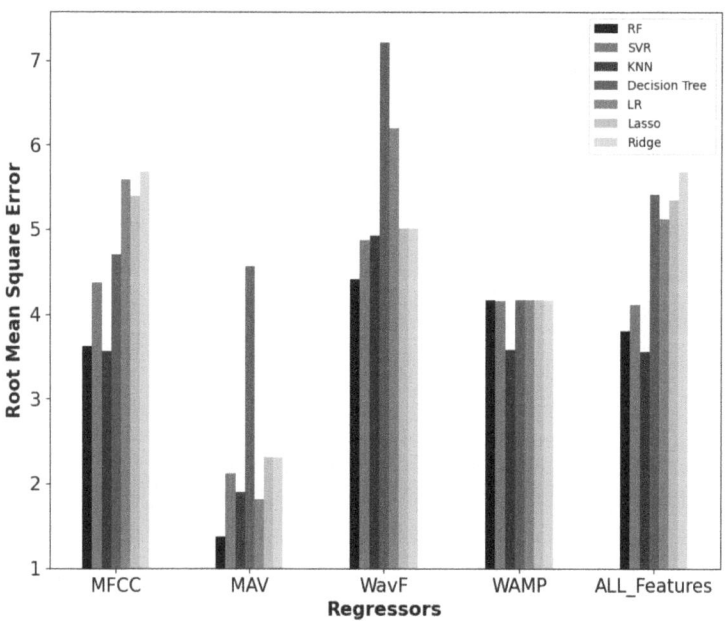

Fig. 3. The bar plot with the root mean square error for the seven regressors with the features using the Suprahyoid [20].

Using global regressors, the RMSE of the suprahyoid was (8.42 ± 1.4 ml), not significantly lower than the infrahyoid channels (9.07 ± 1.9 ml) and all four channels (10.9 ± 2.7 ml). There was no statistical difference between global regressors, with SVR (6.04 ± 1.7 ml) and RF (6.04 ± 1.6 ml) performing better than the others.

The mean performance of each feature, in ascending order, were 6.03 ±1.7 ml for MFCC, 6.04 ± 1.7 ml for Wamp, 6.12 ± 1.65 ml for all features combined, 6.35 ± 1.3

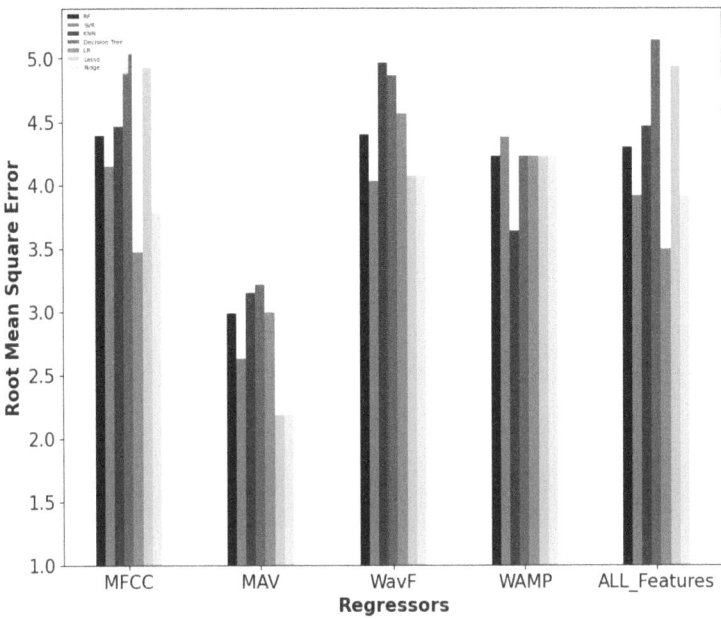

Fig. 4. The bar plot with the root mean square error for the seven regressors with the features using the Infrahyoid Muscles [20].

Table 2. Final Results for the Best Regression Model (RF) using Mean Absolute Volume Feature [20].

Subjects	Average Sip Volume (ml)	RMSE (ml)	Percentage error (%)
S1	19.42 ± 5.00	1.07 ± 1.67	5
S2	8.72 ± 2.95	1.42 ± 0.98	16
S3	12.18 ± 4.19	0.82 ± 1.4	6
S4	11.4 ± 3.59	2.99 ± 1.19	26
S5	18.71 ± 5.94	0.13 ± 1.98	1
S6	12.72 ± 3.85	1.85 ± 1.28	14
S7	21.32 ± 8.47	0.39 ± 2.82	2
S8	13.66 ± 3.15	0.29 ± 1.05	2
S9	7.14 ± 2.86	3.35 ± 0.95	47
Average	13.91 ± 1.27	1.37 ± 0.39	13.22

ml for MAV, 6.46 ± 1.75 ml for WL as indicated in Table 3. There is neither interaction between regressors nor between features. Single-channel investigation showed no difference between channels nor their combinations (infrahyoid and suprahyoid) while using the global regressors. Figure 6 depicts the relationship between the RMSE of the fold and the best result of the global regressors and features of the suprahyoid muscles.

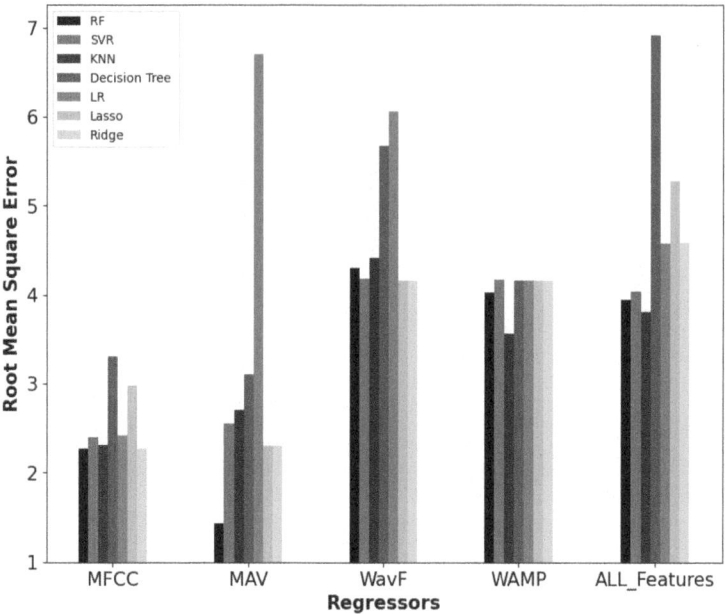

Fig. 5. The bar plot with the root mean square error for the seven regressors with the features using the Infrahyoid Muscles and the Suprahyoid muscles [20].

Figure 7 depicts the relationship between the RMSE of the global regressors' best fold and infrahyoid muscles' features. In contrast, Fig. 8 depicts the relationship between the RMSE of the average ten folds and features of the suprahyoid muscles. Figure 9 depicts the relationship between the RMSE of the average ten folds and features of the infrahyoid muscles. Figure 10 depicts the relationship between the RMSE of the global regressors' best fold (least k) and features of the infrahyoid and suprahyoid muscles. In contrast, Fig. 11 depicts the relationship between the RMSE of the average ten folds and features of the infrahyoid and suprahyoid muscles.

Table 3. Association between features and best global regressor for different channels.

Features	Four channels	Infrahyoid muscles	Suprahyoid muscles
MFCC	**SVR 6.03 ± 1.7 ml**	SVR 6.2 ± 1.75 ml	SVR 6.51 ± 1.8 ml
MAV	SVR 6.35 ± 1.7 ml	SVR 6.54 ± 1.8 ml	SVR 6.51 ± 1.8 ml
WAMP	SVR 6.52 ± 1.8 ml	RF 6.04 ± 1.7 ml	SVR 6.35 ± 1.6 ml
WL	SVR 6.51 ± 1.8 ml	SVR 6.52 ± 1.8 ml	SVR 6.46 ± 1.75 ml
ALL	SVR 6.12 ± 1.65 ml	RF 6.04 ± 1.7 ml	SVR 6.51 ± 1.8 ml

Estimation of Fluid Intake Volume from Surface Electromyography Signals 33

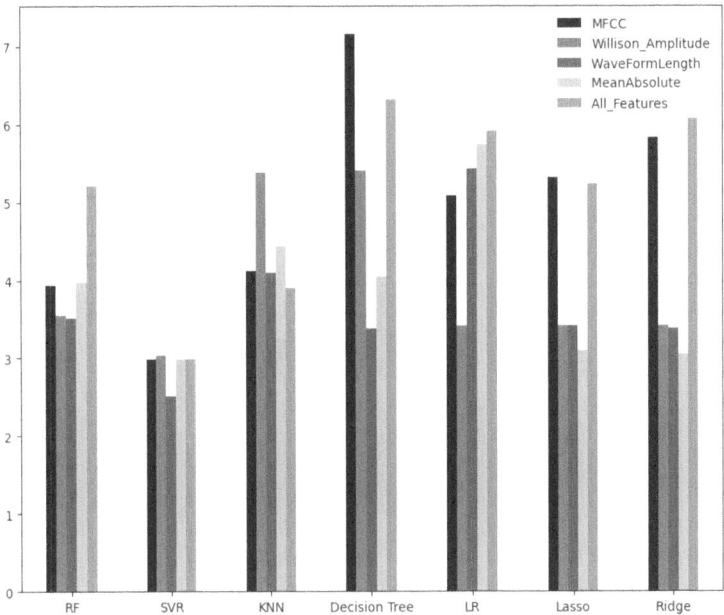

Fig. 6. The bar plot with the RMSE of the fold with the best result of the global seven regressors and the features using the Suprahyoid Muscles.

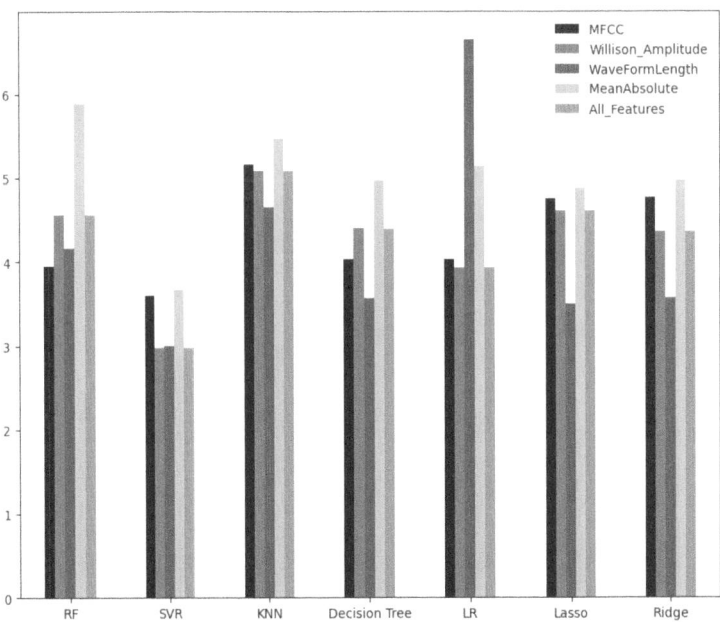

Fig. 7. The bar plot with the RMSE of the fold with the best result of the global seven regressors with the features using the Infrahyoid Muscles.

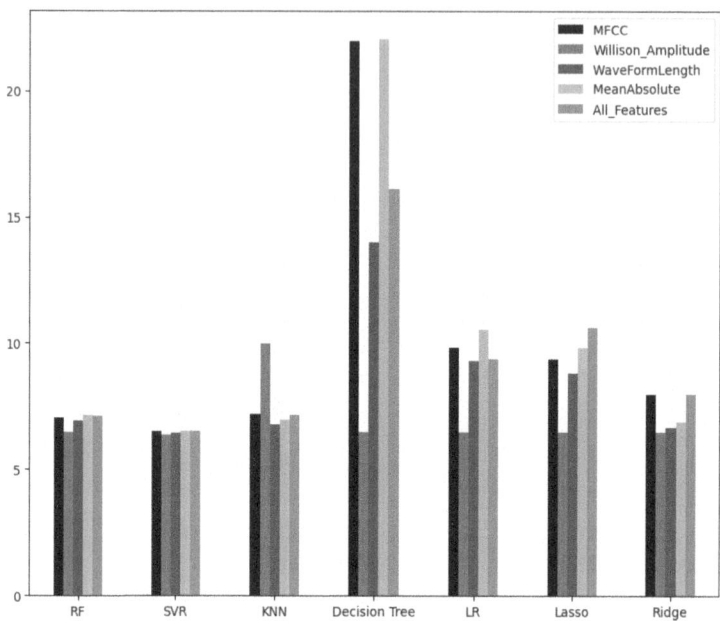

Fig. 8. The bar plot with the RMSE of the average ten folds of the seven global regressors and features using the Suprahyoid Muscles.

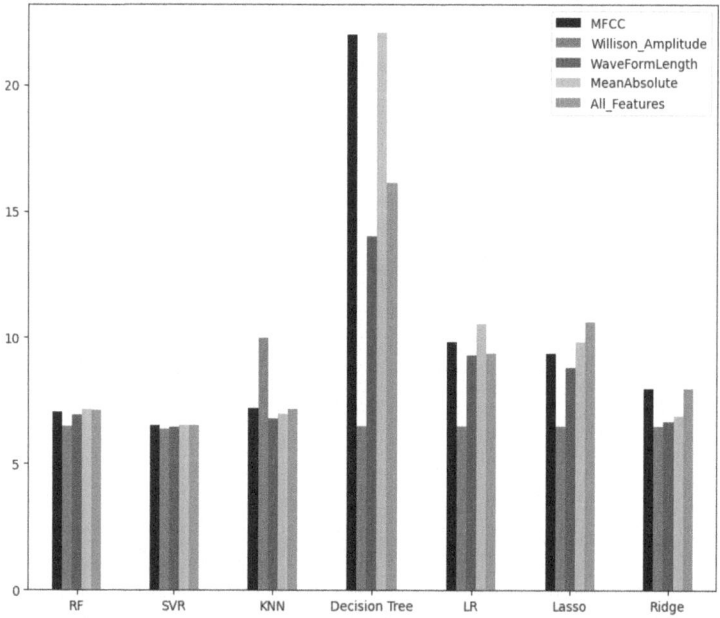

Fig. 9. The bar plot with the RMSE of the average ten folds of the seven global regressors and features using the Infrahyoid Muscles.

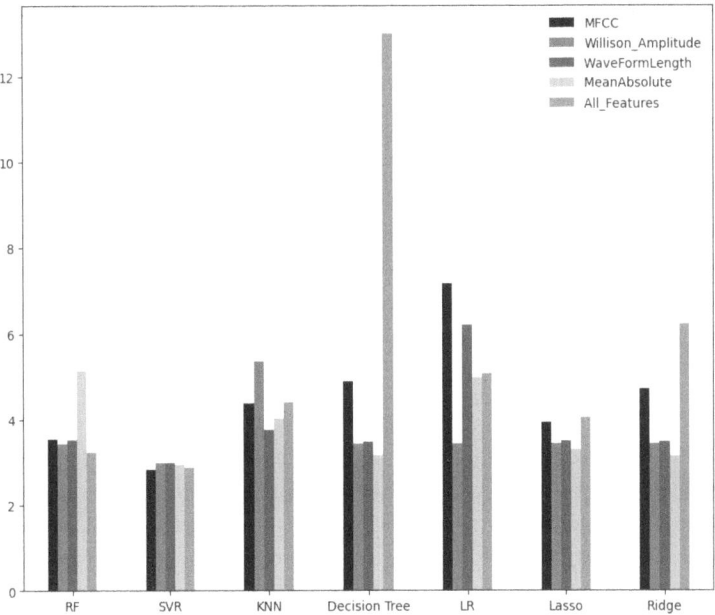

Fig. 10. The bar plot with the RMSE of the fold with the best result of the global seven regressors and features using the Suprahyoid and Infrahyoid Muscles.

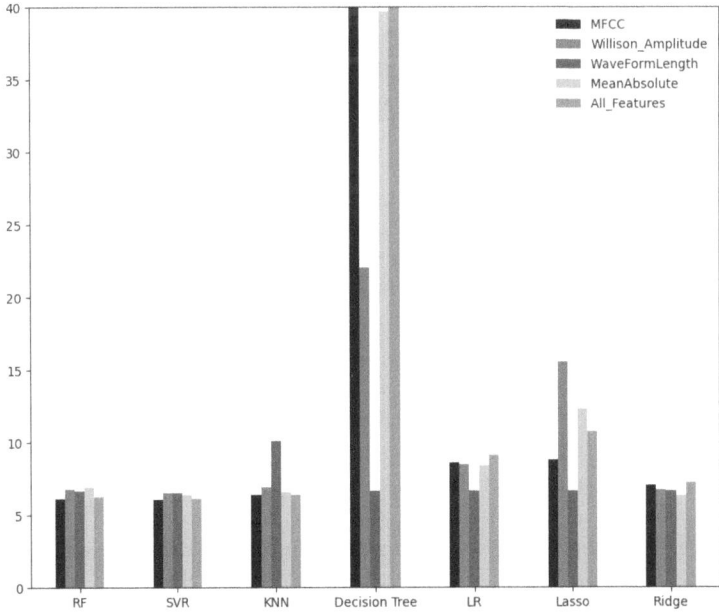

Fig. 11. The bar plot with the RMSE of the average ten folds of the seven global regressors and features using the Suprahyoid and Infrahyoid Muscles.

4 Discussion

This study aimed to compare the power of various regressor techniques in estimating fluid intake volume using surface Electromyographic (sEMG) sensors. The study's regression findings strongly suggest that the estimation of fluid intake volume is feasible using surface EMG. This study demonstrated how regression performance differed depending on whether signals came from the upper two muscles (Suprahyoid muscles), the lower two muscles (Infrahyoid muscles), or all the muscles. We found that solely employing suprahyoid muscles did not produce significantly superior results to those of the infrahyoid muscles. The seven regression models were run on each feature individually and then on all four features collectively to select the best features. This demonstrated that no single regressor works best for all features and that the regressor depends on the feature. There was a significant difference between the regressors. For example, the Random Forest regressor performs best using the Mean Absolute Value feature. Except for the Willison amplitude and MFCC features, statistical analysis did reveal significant variation in how different regressors performed with various features.

Therefore, a single characteristic can be advantageous since it will decrease computing costs and time, particularly for online jobs. Using single channels of the infrahyoid or the suprahyoid muscles or combining a single channel of each to estimate the volume has not improved the results of RMSE. However, the error difference was not too high, indicating that single EMG channels may be used to record the intake data. As a result, in a subsequent study, single channels will be used to record the intake data and investigate whether the fluid estimation performance will be improved. This study also compared subject-specific and global regression techniques. The global regressors were used to estimate the fluid intake volume across all subjects. Although the specific-subject regressors gave RMSE less than global regressors, the performance difference was not very high when considering the best fold. Therefore, their performance can be improved by increasing the sample size and tuning regressors based on artificial neural networks. They are important because of their capability to capture overall trends, patterns, or relationships common to the entire dataset. When used as a global regressor, SVR performed better with MFCC and Willison Amplitude features, while RF performed better with the Mean Absolute Value feature as a subject-specific feature.

The number of studies measuring fluid volume using sEMG is very limited. Kobayashi et al. used a throat microphone to estimate the liquid volume with an RMSE value of 3.33 ml [26]. Malvuccio also estimated the fluid volume consumed using sEMG recordings of individual and continuous swallows, but her work had an RMSE greater than ours [6]. Reducing the error further would be advantageous, so our forthcoming research should include a larger sample size with advanced techniques. Ismail and Kamavuako estimated the fluid intake volume using sEMG with only specific-subject regressors and achieved an RMSE of 1.37 ± 1.1 mL, using only a single feature [20]. However, this paper compares using the subject-specific and global regressors in measuring the fluid volume. In the previous study [20], the Mean Absolute Value (MAV) was the best average feature for measuring fluid intake volume. However, in this study, the performance of using MFCC with the global regressors was better than that of using the MAV. Ismail and Kamavuako have tried to estimate the fluid intake volume by imposing the fluid volume from (5 to 25 ml) which gave poorer results than this study [28]. According to that study, the best procedure for fluid volume estimation is to let the subject drink according to his/her ability, not to force the subject to drink specific volumes, as this will make the subject drink unnaturally, which might affect muscle activation [28].

Although the sEMG performance in estimating fluid intake volume has shown encouraging results compared to other approaches, further validation of these data is necessary. Increasing the sample size is very necessary for the future study to improve the outcomes and model performance. Additionally, the test volunteers must be older adults since their swallowing habits change as people age, which may impact the system's functionality. Finding out if the performance would be affected by age and by increasing the number of subjects is required because this study only used a small number of participants. This study did not consider other variables that could impact the sip volume, such as the liquid temperature and composition. These factors may cause the sip volumes to differ subject to subject, compromising the fluid intake volume technique's estimation ability. Finally, utilizing EMG for fluid monitoring and volume estimation stands out as a promising approach in comparison to other methods identified in the literature review. This is primarily attributed to its non-intrusive, lightweight, and portable sensor and the encouraging results demonstrated in the studies referenced.

5 Conclusion

We have compared for the first time the capability of various regressors to estimate fluid intake from sEMG signals recorded during swallowing events. The results of utilizing only the suprahyoid or infrahyoid muscles did not differ statistically; however, there were statistical differences between the various regressors. RF and SVR regressors were the best ones using the Mean Absolute Value feature in estimating the fluid volume with the lowest error as a subject-specific regressor. However, using the waveform length feature, SVR performed the best as a global regressor. Furthermore, there is an indication that regressor performance is feature-dependent. This outcome is a step forward in using sEMG for hydration monitoring. Further research is needed to investigate using single EMG channels to record more data and estimate the fluid data. We plan for our system to work on infrahyoid muscles for regression and classification.

References

1. El-Sharkawy, A.M., Sahota, O., Maughan, R.J., Lobo, D.N.: The pathophysiology of fluid and electrolyte balance in the older adult surgical patient. Clin. Nutr. **33**(1), 6–13 (2014)
2. Cohen, R., Fernie, G., Fekr, A.R.: Fluid intake monitoring systems for the elderly: a review of the literature. Nutrients **13**, 2092 (2021)
3. Jéquier, E., Constant, F.: Water as an essential nutrient: the physiological basis of hydration. Eur. J. Clin. Nutr. **64**, 115–123 (2010). https://doi.org/10.1038/ejcn.2009.111
4. Lavizzo-Mourey, R.J.: Dehydration in the elderly: a short review. J. Natl. Med. Assoc. **79**, 1033–1038 (1987)
5. Alcorn, E.: Improving fluid balance charts through staff education on a general medical ward: a quality improvement project. Future Healthc. J. **9**, 114 (2022)

6. Malvuccio, C., Kamavuako, E.N.: Detection of swallowing events and fluid intake volume estimation from surface electromyog- raphy signals. In: Proceedings of the 2020 IEEE-EMBS Conference on Biomedical Engineering and Sciences (IECBES), Langkawi Island, Malaysia, 1–3 March 2021, pp. 245–250 (2021)
7. Asogan, H., Raoof, A.: Education and training as key drivers for improving the quality of fluid balance charts: findings from a quality improvement project. BMJ Open Qual. **10**, e001137 (2021)
8. Huhn, S., et al.: The impact of wearable technologies in health research: scoping review. JMIR Mhealth Uhealth **10**, e34384 (2022)
9. Eskandari, S.: Bite detection and differentiation using templates of wrist motion. Master's thesis, Clemson University, Clemson, SC, USA (2013)
10. Liu, K.-C., Hsieh, C.-Y., Huang, H.-Y., Chiu, L.-T., Hsu, S.J.-P., Chan, C.-T.: Drinking event detection and episode identification using 3D-printed smart cup. IEEE Sens. J. **20**, 13743–13751 (2020)
11. Gomes, D., Sousa, I.: Real-time drink trigger detection in free-living conditions using inertial sensors. Sensors **19**, 2145 (2019)
12. Flutura, S., et al.: DrinkWatch: a mobile wellbeing application based on interactive and cooperative machine learning. In: Proceedings of the 2018 International Conference on Digital Health, Lyon, France, 23–26 April 2018. ACM, New York (2018)
13. Ren, Y., Tan, S., Zhang, L., Wang, Z., Yang, J.: Liquid level sensing using commodity WiFi-ina smart home environment. Proc. Interact. Mob. Wearable Ubiquitous Technol. Arch. **4**, 1–30 (2020)
14. Fan, M., Truong, K.N.: SoQr: sonically quantifying the content level inside containers. In: Proceedings of the 2015 ACM International Joint Conference on Pervasive and Ubiquitous Computing-UbiComp 2015, Osaka, Japan, 7–11 September 2015, pp. 3–14. ACM Press, New York (2015)
15. Amft, O., Bannach, D., Pirkl, G., Kreil, M., Lukowicz, P.: Towards wearable sensing-based assessment of fluid intake. In: Proceedings of the 2010 8th IEEE International Conference on Pervasive Computing and Communications Workshops (PERCOM Workshops), Mannheim, Germany, 29 March–2 April 2010, pp. 298–303 (2010)
16. Wellnitz, A., Wolff, J.P., Haubelt, C., Kirste, T.: Fluid intake recognition using inertial sensors. In: Proceedings of the 6th International Workshop on Sensor-Based Activity Recognition and Interaction, pp. 1–7 (2019)
17. Dong, B., Biswas, S.: Meal-time and duration monitoring using wearable sensors. Biomed. Signal Process. Control **32**, 97–109 (2017)
18. Cheng, J., Amft, O., Lukowicz, P.: Active capacitive sensing: exploring a new wearable sensing modality for activity recognition. In: Floréen, P., Krüger, A., Spasojevic, M. (eds.) Pervasive 2010. LNCS, vol. 6030, pp. 319–336. Springer, Heidelberg (2010). https://doi.org/10.1007/978-3-642-12654-3_19
19. Malvuccio, C., Kamavuako, E.N.: The effect of EMG features on the classification of swallowing events and the estimation of fluid intake volume. Sensors **22**, 3380 (2022)
20. Ismail, I.A., Kamavuako, E.N.: Estimation of fluid intake volume from surface electromyography signals: a comparative study of seven regression techniques. In: Proceedings of the 16th International Joint Conference on Biomedical Engineering Systems and Technologies (BIOSTEC 2023), Lisbon, Portugal, 16–18 February 2023, vol. 4, pp. 118–124 (2023)
21. Amft, O., Troster, G.: Methods for detection and classification of normal swallowing from muscle activation and sound. In: Proceedings of the 2006 Pervasive Health Conference and Workshops, Innsbruck, Austria, 21 May 2007, pp. 1–10. IEEE, Piscataway (2007)
22. Nicholls, B., et al.: An EMG-based eating behaviour monitoring system with haptic feedback to promote mindful eating. Comput. Biol. Med. **149**, 106068 (2022)

23. Vaiman, M., Segal, S., Eviatar, E.: Surface electromyographic studies of swallowing in normal children, age 4–12 years. Int. J. Pediatr. Otorhinolaryngol. **68**, 65–73 (2004)
24. Nederkoorn, C., Smulders, F.T., Jansen, A.: Recording of swallowing events using electromyography as a non-invasive measurement of salivation. Appetite **33**, 361–369 (1999)
25. Vinyard, C.J., Fiszman, S.: Using electromyography as a research tool in food science. Curr. Opin. Food Sci. **9**, 50–55 (2016)
26. Huang, Q., Wang, W., Zhang, Q.: Your glasses know your diet: dietary monitoring using electromyography sensors. IEEE Internet Things J. **4**, 705–712 (2017)
27. Kobayashi, Y., Mineno, H.: Fluid intake recognition for nursing care support by leveraging swallowing sound. In: IEEE 3rd Global Conference on Consumer Electronics (2014)
28. Ismail, I., Niazi, I.K., Haavik, H., Kamavuako, E.N.: A cross-day analysis of EMG features, classifiers, and regressors for swallowing events detection and fluid intake volume estimation. Sensors **23**(21), 8789 (2023)

Epileptic Seizure Detection and Prediction for Patient Support

Gul Hameed Khan[1(✉)], Nadeem Ahmad Khan[1], Wala Saadeh[2], and Muahammad Awais Bin Altaf[2]

[1] Lahore University of Management Sciences (LUMS), Lahore, Pakistan
{gul.khan,nkhan}@lums.edu.pk
[2] Engineering and Design Department, Western Washington University, Bellingham, WA, USA
{saadehw,altafm}@wwu.edu

Abstract. The identification of epileptic seizure events is acknowledged as one of the most arduous pattern recognition tasks in chronic brain disorders, and has captured considerable interest among researchers. This endeavor has the potential to significantly enhance patients' quality of life in numerous ways, including accident prevention and mitigating the potential harm associated with epileptic seizures. To enhance seizure detection and prediction efficiency, and provide low complexity pre-trained system, this work presents a trainable hybrid approach to identify seizure events. A shallow autoencoder model has been proposed and implemented to obtain sparse representation of the electroencephalogram (EEG) signal segments followed by the traditional machine learning classifier to categorize the EEG data as either ictal, pre-ictal or inter-ictal. To reveal the ability of EEG channels towards identifying these states, individual channel analysis are presented. Using the CHB-MIT scalp EEG dataset, the proposed method outperforms stae of the art and achieves seizure detection sensitivity of 99.3% and seizure onset prediction sensitivity of 98%. Extremely intensive requirements of computing are minimized by employing a shallow model with fewer parameters to compute and store.

Keywords: Autoencoder · Electroencephalogram · EEG classification · Epilepsy · Seizure detection · Seizure prediction · Single channel model

1 Introduction

Epilepsy is a common neurological disorder reported as a second most occurring neural disease of the brain and number of epileptic patients is increasing rapidly over the recent years [1]. Epileptic seizure appears on spur of the moment and characterized by transient and instantaneous abnormal disruption of brain neurons [2]. Epileptic seizures can cause severe upheaval in emotions, behavior, movements and consciousness of patients, and can lead to a severe injury or even death. Premature death rate of these patients is two to three times than that of disease free individuals and it poses a heavy burden on the patients, their families and the society [3].

Scalp electroencephalogram (EEG) serves as a conventional and relatively cost effective modality for diagnosing epilepsy and detecting and predicting seizures [4].

Automation in this regard is of help both to the neurologists and the patient. Typically, neurologists rely on visually analyzing EEG signals to identify seizures events [5]. However, this process is laborious as it demands neurology professionals to visually assess lengthy EEG recordings. Moreover, identifying epileptic seizure patterns from EEG data poses a significant burden on physicians and introduces the risk of human error [5]. Continuous monitoring of epileptic patients holds significance in preventing severe consequences resulting from seizures. Consequently, the integration of wearable EEG devices with algorithms for predicting and detecting epileptic seizures holds great value in health management systems for patients with chronic diseases. To ensure accurate detection and prediction of seizures it is essential to develop efficient algorithms that can capture brain abnormalities associated with the epileptic seizures in scalp EEG signals [4].

The task of identifying brain abnormalities in EEG data involves distinguishing wave complexes that differentiate normal activities from abnormal ones. The challenge of identifying epileptic episodes in EEG data focuses on recognizing the pre-ictal state (prior to a seizure) for seizure prediction in EEG signals. On the other hand, the seizure detection problem involves discriminating between the ictal state (during a seizure) and the inter-ictal state (normal brain activity) [6]. Early prediction of epileptic seizures allows for adequate time before the actual seizure occurs, which is crucial as timely treatment can prevent the additional harm to epileptic patient. Seizure prediction (or forecasting) entails detecting seizure symptoms and determining whether the patient is on the brink of experiencing a seizure attack [7].

In one of our earlier initiatives related to EEG data presented in [8] we have researched at and published our work on an Intelligent Neurologist Support System, *i-NSS*. In this project we focused on a joint task of seizure detection and marking in Epileptic EEG data along with data reduction and compression for storing EEG data. We explored the synergy in signal processing for these two tasks. Discrete Wavelet Transform (DWT) coefficients are calculated for each epoch and utilized both for classification and compression tasks. Classification is based on computing the statistical features from these DWT coefficients.

The direction of our current project is to investigate methods and systems for analyzing and processing EEG data that are of help in epileptic patient homecare services. The focus in this initiative is both seizure detection and seizure prediction. Portable and wearable devices are central in such services as the patients are ambulatory. This calls for investigating computing efficient algorithms and exploiting synergy in EEG data processing. To this end we have been investigating effective and computing efficient alternates to complex feature extraction methods as was also utilized in our earlier works. In [9] we showed the effectiveness of code generated by a shallow (one-layer) autoencoder (AE) for an EEG epoch in detecting epileptic seizures. Traditional (non-neural) classifiers were experimented with for classification of a single epoch of a single channel EEG and was shown to yield a high accuracy system. On the same lines using the coded representation produced by a shallow AE we designed, trained and tested a seizure prediction algorithm and reported its initial results in [10]. In this article we will present further results of testing our prediction algorithm and its analysis. Like in *i-NSS*, our approach is based on single-channel analysis and can be scaled up to multiple channels, a subject of our ongoing work. It is foreseen that the success of ambulatory patient monitoring hinges upon keeping this number limited to a few key channels as per neurologist patient-specific prior investigation. Our recent work on a wearable sensor that process few EEG channels in the same device [12] is based on such considerations.

In this work we will first provide a short literature review on seizure detection and prediction. This is followed by describing our approaches and techniques involved in seizure detection and prediction Extensive experimental results are provided next. This is followed by a short discussion comparing and analyzing the performance of our approach with the state-of-the-art reported approaches. Final conclusions are drawn at the end of this article.

2 Literature Review

In the existing literature, numerous algorithms have been suggested for classifying EEG data into three categories: ictal, inter-ictal, or pre-ictal. These approaches can be classified into two primary aspects: traditional classification methods that utilize conventional machine learning algorithms to compute statistical features, and deep learning models.

2.1 Traditional Methods

Numerous techniques have been suggested in existing literature to identify seizure events, relying on feature extraction and classification. Machine learning methods and computational algorithms are employed, along with diverse feature extraction techniques, to identify epileptic seizures events from EEG readings. For instance, in a study by [14], empirical mode decomposition (EMD) was utilized for pre-processing of EEG data. Time and frequency domain information was retreived and used to train the classifier model for seizure prediction. Pre-processing of raw EEG such as fast Fourier transform (FFT) is also implemented by some authors to obtain improved classification results for seizure detection [4]. Data pre-processing is used to eliminate noise and artifacts, data transformation, and spectral representation [26]. A Min-Max histogram feature extraction method from EEG data for seizure detection is proposed in [4]. A patient-specific approach that predicts epileptic seizures by applying the common spatial pattern (CSP) feature extraction technique to scalp EEG signals is presented in [17]. Another proposal by [18] introduces a seizure prediction framework that utilizes bag-of-wave (BoWav) feature extraction and synchronization patterns. Spectral and temporal features computation using scattering transform and discrete wavelet transforms (DWT) are also addressed for seizure detection [37]. Dictionary based approaches such as dynamic mode decomposition (DMD) have also been proposed in the literature for seizure detection [15,16]. Other feature extraction methods such as vision transformer [24] and phase lock value (PLV) [31] have also been proposed in the literature for seizure prediction. However, the computation and selection of conventional features is often based on empirical decision-making within a short time frame of EEG signal, which may result in overlooking some key characteristics of EEG data [18]. Due to highly random nature of EEG data, statistical features are not effective representatives of the EEG signal and may lead to miss out the non-stationary property in epileptic EEGs and produce a suboptimal recognition. Moreover, these features require intensive calculations and resources which are not feasible for developing wearable devices.

2.2 Deep Learning Methods

Deep learning algorithms are currently being employed in medical image and signal processing, representing a relatively recent trend. Deep learning-based models do not necessitate handcrafted feature extraction or even pre-processing. These methods automatically select the most representative features of the input data. The robust learning capability of these algorithms has generated considerable interest, made possible by advancements in computing power and the availability of large-scale data. These algorithms hold significant potential and can make a substantial impact, often surpassing the performance achievable by traditional machine learning techniques. Within the field of seizure detection and prediction, convolutional neural networks (CNNs) have gained the majority of researchers' attention [23, 34]. This preference can be attributed to the extensive use of CNNs in signal processing, making them more widely recognized and established within the research community. These methodologies apply data pre-processing or use raw EEG data directly for model training [38]. Detection of epileptic seizures using Quantized deep neural networks (QDNNs) for low-power embedded applications are also developed [39]. A generative model to synthesize EEG data for epileptic seizure prediction using generative adversarial network (GAN) is proposed in [22]. Additionally, Long Short-Term Memory (LSTM) [25], Bi-LSTM [28], graph neural networks (GNN) [29], stacked autoencoders (SAE) [35], and convolutional autoencoders (CAE) have been developed to classify EEG data, resulting in highly accurate systems [7]. Decision fusion of different deep neural network models is also proposed in [20]. A multi-view CNN with consistency-based training strategy for epileptic seizure prediction was proposed in [26]. This strategy makes the model more complex and classification performance is also a major concern to address. However, neural network models usually have numerous arithmetic operations resulting in high computational cost [19]. It is important to note that these methods come with substantial energy consumption and require a large number of parameters to process and hardware resources [19]. The implementation feasibility of deep learning models in energy constrained hardware devices is often overlooked in most contemporary algorithms for epileptic seizure prediction. Consequently, employing these techniques in small, low-power wearable, or implantable medical devices is not feasible. Real-time operation is essential for continuously updating epileptic patients using these devices.

3 Proposed Methodology

Most of the existing approaches employ multiple channels of EEG to extract a group feature vector and label the EEG epoch as seizure (ictal) or non-seizure (non-ictal). Such an approach does not localize evidence of abnormal wave complexes to channel level. Hence, a neurologist has to accomplish this on its own to accept or reject the automatic classification result. In our work on seizure detection and prediction we have followed the approach of analyzing single EEG channel with high accuracy. An approach based on processing a channel individually also has a better potential to be scalable with respect to the number of the channels allowing its deployment in devices using one, few or all EEG channels. For a multi-channel detection this will mean processing the given channels separately as proposed and then ensambling the individual detection

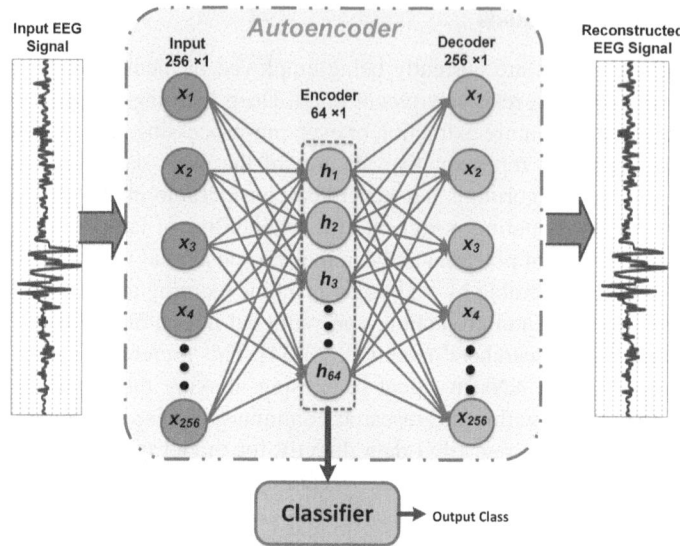

Fig. 1. Work flow architecture of the proposed method [10].

results for a final global decision. This, however, is not discussed in this work. Furthermore, the scope of the current work is limited to achieve low algorithmic computational complexity but does not cover hardware implementation. This could be undertaken in future.

We utilize a coded representation of EEG signal epoch using a neural approach instead of employing some conventional feature extraction method. The utilization of autoencoder (AE), a neural method, has been shown to be highly successful in generating a meaningful low dimensionality coded representation for high-dimensional data just based on minimizing the signal reconstruction loss [35].

For classification we have experimented with multiple conventional classifiers. Hence our approaches for epileptic seizure detection and prediction can be regarded as hybrids of neural and non-neural approaches.

The primary processing architecture for identifying epileptic seizure events is illustrated in Fig. 1. The EEG data is segmented into 1-s intervals for each channel. Previous seizure prediction methods commonly utilize EEG data segments ranging from 1 to 30 s in duration [35]. The EEG dataset utilized in this research has undergone preprocessing steps to remove noise and artifacts. Consequently, computational burden of pre-processing need not to be borne and we directly employ the raw EEG data.

The AE with a single hidden layer processes each 1-s EEG segment to generate its sparse representation. During the training phase, an encoder is employed to derive the sparse representation of the signal, while a decoder is utilized to reconstruct the signal to its original form. Weights and biases of the model are calculated over signal reconstruction error instead of classification results. The sparse signal samples are then used as input to a classifier model to classify the data as either ictal, inter-ictal or pre-ictal.

However, during the testing phase, the decoder component of the AE is omitted, and only the encoder is utilized to obtain sparse representation. Multiple AE Hidden sizes are examined to determine the optimal sparse signal samples capable of accurately classifying the data. As elaborated in the following sections, our core experiment typically uses the AE Hidden size of 64. This corresponds to compress the data from its original length to 64 samples only.

After obtaining the most effective sparse representation of the raw EEG data, we proceed with classification using machine learning algorithms. The sparse signal samples are employed as input for the classifier, enabling seizure detection and prediction in EEG data.

Further details of the tools utilized in this work are explained below:

3.1 Shallow Sparse Autoencoder

An AE consists of two main components: an encoder and a decoder. The decoder aims to minimize the difference between the original dataset x and its reconstructed version $\hat{x}$, as illustrated in Fig. 1. The encoder takes the input x and transforms it into a reduced (low dimensional) representation y containing n samples. Formally, the encoder is a function $f(.)$ that maps the input x to an unknown representation y.

A shallow AE is constructed, comprising a single hidden layer with n neurons in the input/output layer and m neurons in the hidden layer, with $m < n$ as shown in Fig. 1. The encoder layer utilizes shared weights $W^E \in \mathbb{R}^{n \times m}$ and bias vector $b_x \in \mathbb{R}^m$. The decoder layer reconstructs the signal using weights $W^D \in \mathbb{R}^{m \times n}$ and bias vector $b_y \in \mathbb{R}^n$. The weights and biases of the model are updated based on the signal reconstruction error rather than classification results. The scaled conjugate gradient (SCG) algorithm is employed to update these weight and bias values.

The encoding process for an input EEG signal $x \in \mathbb{R}^n$ can be formulated as follows:

$$y - f(W^E x + b_x) \tag{1}$$

where $f(\cdot)$ represents the activation function in the encoder neurons. Two inputs, a bias vector b and a matrix W, are used to configure the decoder. In most cases, the activation function is selected based on the characteristics of the available data [35]. However, in contrast to non-linear functions, linear activation helps in building a system with low computational cost. For this reason, both the encoding and decoding procedures will use linear activations. For the encoder's activation function, the saturating linear transfer function (Satlin) is described as:

$$satlin(x) = \begin{cases} -1 & x < -1 \\ 0 & -1 \leqslant x \leqslant 1 \\ 1 & x > 1 \end{cases} \tag{2}$$

Finding the values of the training parameters $\theta = (W, b_x, b_y)$ that minimize the reconstruction loss for a given dataset is the goal of AE training.

$$\Theta = min_\theta L(x, \hat{x}) = min_\theta L(x, f(W^T x + b)) \tag{3}$$

The reconstruction loss L in AE's training phase is typically derived from the square of the error:

$$L(\theta) = \frac{1}{n}\sum_{k=1}^{n}(x - \hat{x})^2 \quad (4)$$

Here, both the n and m represents the number of samples in the signal. The decoder layer reconstructs the sparse vector $y \in \mathbb{R}^m$ to its original form as:

$$\hat{x} = W^D y + b_y \quad (5)$$

AE's objective function reconstructs the input to its original form. High weights of hidden layers make the generated features more dependent on the network structure rather than the input data. Therefore, to avoid this complexity, sparse AE imposes weight-decay regularization so as to keep neuron weights small.

$$\Theta = \alpha min_\theta L(x, \hat{x}) + \lambda ||W||^2 \quad (6)$$

Here, α is the scale parameter to control the weights of the data reconstruction loss. We used L_2 regularization $||W||^2$ to ensure weight matrix W having small elements. Hyper parameter λ is incorporated to control the regularization strength. Transfer function to compute decoder layer's output is linear function (Purelin) $f(x) = x$. These functions are applied to each signal sample using the Mean Square Error (MSE) loss function, presented in Eq. 4. MSE is used in the AE's training phase to compare the original and reconstructed signals. Encoding yields a sparse representation of the signal, while decoding generates a reconstruction of the signal to its original form. The decoding is only added in training phase to ensure the best sparse representation of the data possible.

Sparsity level of the AE for input signal of length n and hidden size m is given as:

$$SparsityLevel = \frac{n}{m} \quad (7)$$

3.2 Classifiers

We experimented with various machine learning algorithms for classification of the EEG data such as k nearest neighbour (kNN), support vector machine (SVM), quadratic discriminant analysis (QDA), decision tree (DT), naive bayes (NB) and Softmax layer. kNN classifier achieved the highest classification results for seizure detection among all the mentioned classifier models. For seizure prediction, SVM stands at top of the list. Further implementation details of these classifiers is discussed below.

SVM. In this work, we employed a Gaussian Support Vector Machine (SVM) classifier for identifying the seizure events. The Gaussian kernel SVM is widely used and recognized as one of the most effective techniques for supervised learning due to its excellent performance [43]. To ensure optimal model performance, it is crucial to accurately determine hyperparameters such as the kernel width and penalty factor.

To thoroughly evaluate the performance of the Gaussian kernel SVM, we conducted a comprehensive analysis where hyperparameters were set to their extreme values (either 0 or infinity) as discussed in [43]. Furthermore, the choice of kernel function significantly impacts the characteristics of the SVM [43]. In our approach, we utilized the Gaussian kernel as shown in Eq. 8. By setting the kernel scale to 4 and the kernel offset to 0.1, we generated an optimized hyperplane in the kernel space. These parameter values ensured that the training instances were separable and led to optimal results. It's important to note that the feature space to which the training data is mapped is determined by the kernel width, which greatly influences the training procedure's accuracy and success.

$$k(x_i, x_j) = exp(-\frac{||x_i - x_j||^2}{2\sigma^2}) \tag{8}$$

Although, the study in [43] experimented with LOO method, however, we use 10-fold cross validation (CV) instead due to the fact that LOO is computationally very high as compared to k-fold CV.

kNN. To distinguish between ictal and inter-ictal EEG data, a weighted k-nearest neighbors (kNN) classifier has been employed. To minimize the computational burden of the classification algorithm, we have chosen to select 10 nearest neighbors for the kNN approach. An important consideration for the kNN classifier's performance is the selection of the hyperparameter k. Opting for a very small k value would increase sensitivity to outliers, while a larger k value might incorporate features from other classes into the neighborhood. To address these uncertain conditions, we have opted for a weighted kNN approach. The weight kernel chosen to handle this uncertainty is the 'squared inverse distance,' where the value decreases as the distance increases. The Euclidean distance metric is used to determine the neighboring data points for the kNN process. In order to handle uncertain outliers and account for incomplete and inconsistent information within the features, an 'exhaustive neutrosophic' set has been utilized to establish the decision criteria [18]. Furthermore, if multiple classes have the same smallest cost, the label is assigned to the class with the smallest index.

QDA. QDA is a variation of Linear Discriminant Analysis(LDA) that differs in its assumption about the covariance matrix of the classes. Unlike LDA, QDA does not assume that the classes share the same covariance matrix. Instead, it allows each class to have its own covariance matrix. As a result, the decision boundary between classes in QDA is a quadratic surface, in contrast to the linear hyperplane in LDA.

DT. According to [45], DT is considered the least computationally intensive classifier. In our implementation, we employ an 'exact search' algorithm with a tree consisting of 159 nodes to determine the optimal split. The split criterion used is 'gdi' (Gini impurity).

NB. NB is a classification algorithm that relies on Bayes' theorem, which is derived from conditional probability theory, and makes an assumption of independence among predictors [3]. In other words, the NB classifier assumes that the presence of a specific feature in a class is independent of the presence of other features. For our implementation, we utilized the Gaussian kernel function with a normal distribution for this classifier.

Softmax. The Softmax layer is commonly employed as the final layer in neural networks designed for data classification [38]. In our approach, we train the Softmax layer using the same methodology as the previously mentioned classifiers. The 'binary cross entropy' function is used with the SCG algorithm to update the weight and bias values.

4 Evaluation Data

To assess the efficacy of the proposed method, we conducted experiments using the CHB-MIT PhysioNet scalp EEG database, which was collected from the Children's Hospital Boston [44]. The database consists of 916 h of continuous scalp EEG (sEEG) monitoring, encompassing 163 seizure occurrences from 23 pediatric patients. The recordings from 22 participants were organized into 23 cases and were sampled at a frequency of 256 Hz.

We evaluate the common 18 channels for each patient to ensure model consistency and patient wise uniformity as in [25, 30, 32]. Because there are numerous patients in the experiment using different channels, we used the same 18 channels that all patients had. Therefore, we utilize 18 channels ("FP1-F7", "F7-T7", "T7-P7", "P7-O1", "FP1-F3", "F3-C3", "C3-P3", "P3-O1", "FP2-F4", "F4-C4", "C4-P4", "P4-O2", "FP2-F8", "F8-T8", "T8-P8", "P8-O2", "FZ-CZ", "CZ-PZ"). Table 1 shows the details of the subjects' information selected from the CHB-MIT dataset for seizure prediction task. However, for seizure detection, we utilized the entire CHB-MIT dataset.

Table 1. Subjects information from the CHB-MIT database for seizure prediction [10].

Patient ID	No. of seizure events	Inter-ictal Duration (hrs)
1	7	14
2	3	23
3	6	22
5	5	14
9	4	46
10	6	26
13	5	14
14	5	5
18	6	24
19	3	25
20	5	20
21	4	22
23	5	13
Total	64	268.6

5 Experimental Results

This section evaluates and discusses the classification performance of the proposed model for seizure detection and prediction. We experimented the proposed algorithm with various hidden sizes of the AE. For a an input size of 256, the encoder layer length varies from 64 to 8, corresponding to the sparsity levels 4 to 32 as demonstrated in Eq. 7. Reducing the AE's hidden size will decrease the computational cost of the algorithm. In addition, analyzing the EEG signals towards seizure detection and prediction with different hidden sizes of the AE will help to select an optimum hidden size as we do not have a specific formula to build an AE with the most appropriate hidden size.

The MATLAB 2021 is utilized to implement the proposed algorithm. The experiments are conducted on a system equipped with an Intel Core(TM) i7 processor operating at 3.20 GHz and 24 GB of memory.

Table 2. Average seizure detection results of CHB-MIT database for various AE Hidden sizes with different classifiers [11].

AE Hidden size	Classifier	Accuracy(%)	Sensitivity(%)	Specificity(%)
64	kNN	98.60	95.23	98.90
	SVM	98.38	65.29	99.39
	QDA	87.47	47.63	88.71
	NB	92.83	58.23	93.05
	DT	89.96	39.17	91.05
	Softmax	68.31	51.24	61.70
32	kNN	93.08	94.01	93.09
	SVM	99.29	89.03	99.30
	QDA	80.10	60.09	80.12
	NB	82.38	46.90	82.96
	DT	93.99	43.42	94.07
	Softmax	78.50	73.82	79.98
20	kNN	90.00	93.42	90.00
	SVM	98.17	88.89	98.18
	QDA	86.34	61.35	86.37
	NB	82.36	52.32	83.10
	DT	94.28	43.26	94.36
	Softmax	71.63	53.36	74.10
16	kNN	88.77	91.15	89.36
	SVM	98.10	61.79	99.06
	QDA	90.85	43.10	91.98
	NB	90.52	38.36	91.65
	DT	92.55	35.65	93.79
	Softmax	81.62	42.86	72.60
8	kNN	84.47	94.42	84.45
	SVM	97.24	76.16	97.27
	QDA	92.47	43.57	92.54
	NB	88.06	48.23	88.63
	DT	94.97	35.69	95.06
	Softmax	53.68	58.90	48.86

Table 3. Channel wise average seizure detection results of CHB-MIT database for kNN classifier with AE Hidden size 64 [11].

Channel	AC(%)	Sen(%)	Spe(%)
'FP1F7'	98.17	95.04	98.28
'F7T7'	99.46	94.17	99.46
'T7P7'	96.26	95.15	96.26
'P7O1'	99.32	94.47	99.32
'FP1F3'	98.28	95.20	98.98
'F3C3'	98.60	95.16	98.60
'C3P3'	98.72	95.07	98.72
'P3O1'	99.20	94.59	99.20
'FP2F4'	99.04	95.04	99.04
'F4C4'	99.35	96.39	99.35
'C4P4'	99.21	94.81	99.38
'P4O2'	99.05	96.40	99.05
'FP2F8'	99.90	94.59	99.90
'F8T8'	98.58	95.40	98.58
'T8P8'	98.17	94.47	98.17
'P8O2'	98.85	99.29	98.85
'FZCZ'	98.65	95.46	98.97
'CZPZ'	99.79	94.33	99.79

5.1 Seizure Detection

Experimental Setup. In this study, we utilize approximately 916 h of scalp EEG recordings from the CHB-MIT dataset, which contains a total of 185 seizure events. For the training set, approximately 5 h of recordings (consisting of 1-s duration EEG epochs) are randomly selected, encompassing both seizure and non-seizure events. The seizure and non-seizure ratio is set at 40% and 60% respectively. This choice is motivated by the dataset's characteristic of having extensive EEG recordings with infrequent seizure occurrences. Thus, a balanced ratio of seizure and non-seizure EEG epochs is maintained to ensure effective training on seizure events. The 'mean absolute error' value for signal reconstruction error during AE training is 6.2 for AE Hidden size 64.

For testing the performance of our system, we utilize the remaining 911 h of EEG data. The AE model is trained using the training data to obtain the encoded representation of the input signal. This encoded representation of the EEG epochs is then employed to train the classifier. To mitigate the risk of model overfitting, a 5-fold cross-validation strategy is implemented during AE training. We experimented with various machine learning classifiers for seizure detection and their classification performance is provided in the next section.

Performance Evaluation. Table 2 provides a concise comparison of the results obtained with various classifiers, using the average results across all EEG channels. The average testing measures for accuracy (Ac), sensitivity (Sen), and specificity (Spe) are presented for each classifier model. The kNN classifier demonstrated the highest performance for all three metrics at AE Hidden Size 64, followed by SVM. On the other hand, the traditional Softmax classifier, commonly employed in deep learning models, exhibited the lowest figures among all the listed classifiers.

Seizure detection results across all EEG channels (individually) are presented in Table 3 using kNN. Each channel demonstrates high mean values (exceeding 94%), indicating the effectiveness of the proposed methodology. This finding underscores the capability of the proposed approach to achieve results comparable to previous studies on seizure detection, even when utilizing a single EEG channel. It is important to note that the selection of the channel by a neurologist is a prerequisite for obtaining these results.

5.2 Seizure Prediction

Experimental Setup. Inter-ictal period is defined as the time interval between at least 4 h (hrs) before the start of a seizure and 4 hrs after it has ended [22]. The CHB-MIT dataset reveals that seizures often occur closely together. When predicting seizures, our focus is on forecasting a seizure event that will happen approximately 30 min after the previous one. Hence, we consider seizures that occur within this time-frame as a single seizure, with the start time of the first seizure being considered as the beginning of the combined seizure. Moreover, we only consider patients who have fewer than 10 seizures per day for the prediction task. This exclusion is because there is no need to predict seizure occurrences for patients who experience seizures, on average, every 2 h. Based on these criteria, we have identified 13 participants who possess sufficient data, including a minimum of three primary seizures and three hours of interictal recording. Table 1 provides a comprehensive description of each subject's information, including their subject ID, total number of seizure occurrences, and the length of the inter-ictal period.

The Seizure Prediction Horizon (SPH) represents the time duration between the alert being triggered in anticipation of a seizure and the actual onset of the ictal state. To ensure an accurate prediction, a seizure should occur after the SPH but before the Seizure Occurrence Period (SOP), which indicates the estimated time frame for a seizure to happen. If the prediction algorithm generates a positive signal (indicating an imminent seizure), but no seizure occurs during the SOP, a false alarm is generated. Once the alert has been triggered, the optimal therapeutic use of the SPH is to provide the patient with enough time to take preventive measures. It is crucial for a patient's SPH to be sufficiently long to allow for adequate safety precautions after the alarm is activated. However, it is also important not to make the SOP excessively long in order to ensure the patient's comfort. In this study, we have adopted a SPH period of 10 min and an SOP period of 30 min.

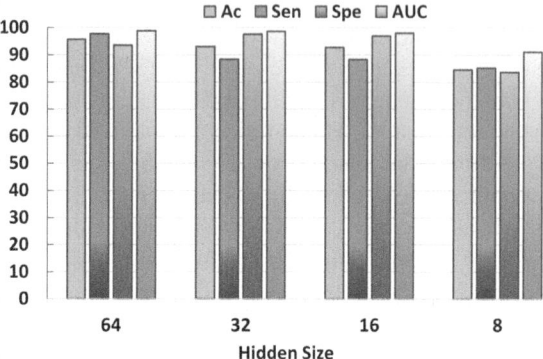

Fig. 2. Variations in Seizure prediction performance of the proposed method using different hidden sizes (Sparsity Levels) of the AE for channel 'FzCz' (best case) [10]

Table 4. Average seizure prediction results for each channel using the AE Hidden size 64.

Channel	Ac(%)	Sen(%)	Spe(%)	AUC(%)
'FZCZ'	**96.0**	**98.0**	**93.0**	**99.0**
'P7O1'	96.0	98.0	94.0	99.0
'FP2F4'	95.0	97.0	94.0	99.0
'P8O2'	94.1	96.8	97.0	97.5
'F7T7'	94.1	89.3	97.0	98.7
'CZPZ'	93.9	90.1	97.3	97.6
'F4C4'	93.7	89.3	97.9	97.1
'F3C3'	93.6	98.2	98.1	94.6
'T7P7'	93.0	86.0	99.0	98.0
'T8P8'	92.1	88.1	96.1	98.0
'C3P3'	92.0	96.5	87.4	91.5
'F8P8'	92.0	89.8	94.1	97.0
'FP1F3'	91.8	96.1	88.5	95.5
'P4O2'	91.8	84.3	97.5	92.4
'P3O1'	91.7	82.5	99.3	92.0
'FP2F8'	91.4	87.1	95.1	96.0
'FP2F4'	91.1	86.2	95.8	96.0
'FP1F7'	**91.1**	**85.8**	**96.2**	**97.0**

Inter-ictal EEG recordings are more common compared to pre-ictal EEG recordings because the occurrence of the ictal state is infrequent during long hours of EEG monitoring. In machine learning methods, it is generally expected that data from different classes should be evenly distributed [22]. If a classifier is trained on a significantly larger number of examples from one class compared to others, it may exhibit bias and favor imbalanced decisions. To address the problem of class imbalance, several strategies have been discussed in the literature, such as the use of overlapping window [23,27], generative adversarial network (GAN) [22], and synthetic minority over-sampling technique (SMOTe) [36]. In our approach, we employ SMOTe during the training phase to generate additional pre-ictal data, effectively mitigating the issue of imbalanced data as outlined in [36].

Using the CHB-MIT database, the AE model for sparse representation of the input signal is trained using 10 min of pre-ictal EEG data (1-s duration segments) for each seizure. For example, as indicated in Table 1, Patient 1 has experienced seven seizures. Therefore, we extract 70 (7×10) minutes of pre-ictal data and the same amount of data for the inter-ictal phase for this patient. Various model assessment strategies have been presented in the literature, including patient-wise data partitioning into train and test sets [28], k-fold CV [22,25], and LOO CV [32]. As a result, for a fair comparison and to avoid over-fitting, we evaluated the performance of the proposed seizure prediction model using the same 10-fold CV as the majority of existing approaches. Raw EEG segments of duration 1 s were utilized without any preprocessing. The compressed form of these segments was utilized to train the 10-fold CV based classifier.

Based on our earlier experiments on seizure detection, we selected only SVM classifier for seizure prediction task. SVM classifier offers less computational complexity and produce close to best results, offering a best compromise. Moreover, since, seizure prediction is applicable in the context of facilitating the patient, we have experimented with patient specific training and testing for this task.

Performance Evaluation. The proposed classification approach is evaluated using an AE with variable hidden sizes that generates sparse signals of varying lengths. Figure 2 illustrates the average Ac, Sen, Spe, and area under the curve (AUC) of the proposed method for seizure prediction at each sparsity level for EEG channel 'FzCz'. Statistical analysis of performance evaluation demonstrates that the proposed classification model can be utilized in a variety of system-required scenarios. The highest sparsity level reported is 32, which corresponds to compressing an input signal of length 256 to merely 8 samples. Based on our earlier results on seizure detection and this experiment in Fig. 2 for seizure prediction, we find the optimal AE Hidden size of value 64 for rest of the experiments.

Table 5. Patient wise seizure prediction results for the best and worst performing channels with AE Hidden size 64 [10]

Patient ID	Channel 'FzCz' (Best Case)				Channel 'FP1F7' (Worst Case)			
	Ac	Sen	Spe	AUC	Ac	Sen	Spe	AUC
1	99.0	100	97.8	100	92.6	89.2	96.1	97.0
2	93.8	98.7	91.8	98.0	89.7	85.8	93.4	94.0
3	96.3	98.1	93.0	99.0	88.0	97.4	78.4	89.0
5	96.1	98.1	95.0	99.0	83.4	74.7	92.2	92.0
9	97.5	98.3	94.6	99.0	89.2	82.4	95.9	90.0
10	95.0	99.3	91.0	100	91.9	86.0	97.8	94.0
13	95.7	99.4	91.8	98.0	88.0	87.2	88.9	94.0
14	94.1	91.2	98.0	99.0	87.2	78.3	96.9	95.0
18	95.4	99.1	91.3	100	86.8	86.5	87.1	88.0
19	94.1	97.0	91.5	98.0	94.0	97.8	90.3	95.0
20	97.0	99.0	96.1	100	97.1	96.0	98.2	95.0
21	95.8	99.3	92.5	99.0	87.1	85.3	88.8	91.0
23	92.0	91.0	92.0	95.0	86.1	84.6	87.7	90.0
Average	96.0	98.0	93.5	98.8	89.3	87.1	92.0	92.6

Among the 18 available EEG channels of the dataset, we present the results of best and worst performing channels. Channel 'FzCz' corresponds to the best case providing the highest average classification results for all the patients, whereas, channel 'FP1F7' is the worst case. Table 5 provides a summary of the patient-specific seizure prediction results achieved with these two channels. Performance metrics include prediction Ac, Sen, Spe, and AUC. Even when using a single EEG channel, the proposed approach can produce results comparable to those of previous studies on the prediction of seizures. The prerequisite is the Neurologist's selection of the channel.

The average seizure prediction performance obtained by the proposed method for each available EEG channel is presented in Table 4. Classification results shown in Table 4 for individual EEG channels are the average of all subjects used in this work and channels are ranked on the basis of their prediction performance. Channel 'FzCz' stands on the top with highest classification performance for both test cases, whereas, channel 'FP1F7' and 'FP2F4' provides the minimum results.

Table 6. Comparison of seizure detection results with state of the art techniques for CHB-MIT database [11].

Ref. - Year	CH	Features	Classifier	Ac (%)	Sen (%)	Spe (%)
[1] - 2020	21	Multiple Spectral and Temporal	CE-stSENet	95.9	92.4	96.0
[3] - 2020	22	30 Statistical features	SVM, kNN and 8 other	86.2	80.3	92.2
[4] - 2020	22	24 Statistical	SVM	94.5	–	–
[41] - 2019	23	SAE	CNN and SVM	92.0	95.0	90.0
[38] - 2019	23	Deep CNN	Dense and SoftMax	98.0	90.0	91.6
[2] - 2019	23	Deep CAE	FC and SoftMax	93.9	–	–
[40] - 2019	22	Statistical and PCA	SVM and Naive Bayes	95.6	95.7	96.5
[5] - 2018	22	Statistical and Morphological	Change Point Detector	–	96.0	–
[13] - 2018	22	FFT and Deep CNN	FC and SoftMax	96.1	–	–
[15] - 2018	23	EMD dictionary	SVM	92.9	94.3	91.5
[42] - 2018	21	Deep CNN	SoftMax	–	87.9	86.5
[37] - 2017	22	FFT, DWT, Scattering Transform	Group Invariant Scattering	–	91.4	86.0
[6] - 2016	23	Poincare and PCA	LDA and Naive Bayes	94.7	89.1	94.8
Proposed (All channels mean)	1	64 Shallow encoded	kNN	**98.6**	**95.2**	**98.9**
Proposed (Channel 'P8O2')	1	64 Shallow encoded	kNN	**98.8**	**99.3**	**98.8**

CH : No. of Channels used;

6 Discussion

In order to demonstrate the effectiveness of the proposed seizure detection method, the obtained results are compared with state-of-the-art approaches using the CHB-MIT dataset, as shown in Table 6. We present the best results achieved using a single EEG channel. The AE utilized a Hidden size of 64. It is important to note that conducting an exact comparison is challenging due to variations in the number of channels used, different training and testing scenarios, training approaches (such as addressing

Table 7. Average classification results comparison with some recent seizure prediction methods for CHB-MIT database [10].

Ref.	Subj.	CH	SL	SPH (min)	Evaluation	Data balancing	Ac (%)	Sen (%)	Spe (%)	AUC (%)
[21]	13	22	5	30	10-fold CV	Overlap window	92.0	87.7	92.8	91.3
[22]	13	22	60	10	10-fold CV	GAN	92.0	90.9	89	–
[23]	13	22	30	30	LOO-CV	Overlap window	–	81.2	–	–
[25]	23	18	10	10	k-fold CV	–	92.6	91.2	94.1	–
[31]	19	23	8	15	Train/Test split	Overlap window	89.9	92.9	87.0	–
[33]	22	23	29	32	k-Fold CV	SMOTe	–	93	92.5	–
[26]	13	All	30	30	LOO-CV	Overlap window	–	88.3	–	–
[27]	24	23	10	60	10-fold CV	Overlap window	91.5	92.4	89.9	96.9
[28]	13	23	5	5	Test 1 patient; Train Rest	–	80.0	–	74.1	–
[30]	17	18	1.5	30	4-fold CV	Overlap window	–	97.1	95.6	91.7
[29]	19	All	5	15	LOO-CV	–	–	95.5 –	–	93.8 –
[32]	16	18	4	30	LOO-CV	Overlap window	–	93.3	–	–
[34]	16	18	10	8	70% Train 30% Test	Overlap window	93.4	–	–	86.5
This work (Channel 'FP1F7', Worst Case)	13	1	1	10	**10-fold CV**	SMOTe	**89.3**	**87.1**	**92.0**	**92.6**
This work (Channel 'FzCz', Best case)	13	1	1	10	**10-fold CV**	SMOTe	**96.0**	**98.0**	**93.5**	**98.8**

CH: No. of Channels used; SL: Segment Length(sec); Subj.: No. of Subjects used imbalanced data), evaluation techniques (LOO, k-fold CV, etc.) and varying EEG epoch sizes among these approaches. To ensure a fair comparative analysis, we employed a framework that is highly relevant to existing high-performance approaches. Nevertheless, Table 6 provides information on different approaches that classify EEG data at the segment level (with intervals ranging from 1 to 30 s) and report classification results in terms of Ac, Sen, and Spe. Both multi-channel and single-channel methods are included in the comparison, and patient-specific results are also indicated.

Table 7 provides a performance comparison between the proposed algorithm and other existing approaches for epileptic seizure prediction using the CHB-MIT dataset. The classification performance statistics demonstrate that our method produces comparable results to the state-of-the-art, particularly in terms of prediction sensitivity, which is a crucial factor in ensuring that no seizure event prediction is missed.

Existing methods in the literature do not extend their analysis to the level of individual channels for seizure prediction and detection. Instead, they only provide an overall assessment based on all available EEG channels. In contrast, the proposed method offers both individual channel assessment and multi-channel evaluations. Furthermore, certain drawbacks can be found in existing methods, such as the inclusion of pre and post-processing units that involve data transformation and noise addition. In the proposed method, these steps are avoided to reduce computational requirements.

Additionally, some approaches employ convolutional layers in their neural network architecture, which can be computationally expensive compared to a fully connected network. On the other hand, the proposed seizure prediction and detection model adopts a shallow architecture instead of deep networks. This choice enhances computational efficiency since the number of network parameters is significantly reduced compared to deep networks.

7 Conclusion

We have proposed and implemented high performance epileptic seizure detection and prediction approaches. In order to acquire a compact but effective representation of the EEG signal, a shallow AE (instead of deep network or traditional complex feature extraction stage) is proposed with only one encoder layer. Relatively low complexity machine learning classifier labels the EEG data (as 1 sec EEG segments) as either ictal, pre-ictal or inter-ictal depending on the task (detection or prediction). Our methodology outperforms the state of the art methods with regard to classification accuracy, sensitivity and specificity with classification accuracy of 99% for seizure detection and 96% for seizure prediction. We have compared the performance with both deep learning and traditional approaches. Unlike the existing multi-channel seizure detection methods in the literature, our approach presents analysis at single channel level. In future we will extend our approach to multi-channel based on ensembling the results of a single channel. Our next goal in this regard is to develop a system which allows compression and decompression of EEG data with low reconstruction loss simultaneously along with ability to classify it.

Acknowledgements. We would like to thank SIVP cluster of EE LUMS for housing this work.

References

1. Li, Y., Liu, Y., Cui, W.G., Guo, Y.Z., Huang, H., Hu, Z.Y.: Epileptic seizure detection in EEG signals using a unified temporal-spectral squeeze-and-excitation network. IEEE Trans. Neural Syst. Rehabil. Eng. **28**(4), 782–794 (2020)
2. Yuan, Y., Xun, G., Jia, K., Zhang, A.: A multi-view deep learning framework for EEG seizure detection. IEEE J. Biomed. Health Inform. **23**, 83–94 (2019)
3. Yang, S., et al.: Selection of features for patient-independent detection of seizure events using scalp EEG signals. Comput. Biol. Med. 119 (2020)
4. Jiang, Z., Zhao, W.: Optimal selection of customized features for implementing seizure detection in wearable electroencephalography sensor. IEEE Sens. J. **20**(21), 12941–12949 (2020)
5. Khanmohammadi, S., Chou, C.A.: Adaptive seizure onset detection framework using a hybrid PCA-CSP approach. IEEE J. Biomed. Health Inform. **22**(1), 154–160 (2018)
6. Zabihi, M., et al.: Analysis of high-dimensional phase space via Poincaré section for patient-specific seizure detection. IEEE Trans. Neural Syst. Rehabil. Eng. **24**, 386–398 (2016)
7. Tăuţan, A.-M., Dogariu, M., Ionescu, B.: Detection of epileptic seizures using unsupervised learning techniques for feature extraction. In: 41st Annual International Conference of the IEEE Engineering in Medicine and Biology Society (EMBC), pp. 2377–2381 (2019)
8. Khan, N.A., Khan, G.H., Ahmad, M.A., Awais bin Altaf, M., Osama Tarar, M.: The extended *i*-NSS: an intelligent EEG tool for diagnosing and managing epilepsy. In: Ye, X., Soares, F., De Maria, E., Gómez Vilda, P., Cabitza, F., Fred, A., Gamboa, H. (eds.) BIOSTEC 2020. CCIS, vol. 1400, pp. 243–262. Springer, Cham (2021). https://doi.org/10.1007/978-3-030-72379-8_12
9. Khan, G.H., et al.: Classifying single channel epileptic EEG data based on sparse representation using shallow autoencoder. In: 43rd Annual International Conference of the IEEE Engineering in Medicine & Biology Society (EMBC), pp. 643–646 (2021)
10. Khan, G.H., Khan, N.A., Saadeh, W., Altaf, M.A.B.: Using sparse representation of EEG signal from a shallow sparse autoencoder for epileptic seizure prediction. In: BIOSIGNALS (2023)
11. Khan, G.H., Khan, N.A., Altaf, M.A.B., Abbasi, Q.: A shallow autoencoder framework for epileptic seizure detection in EEG signals. Sensors **23**(8), 4112 (2023)
12. Sheeraz, M., et al.: Flexible EEG headband with artifact reduction and continuous electrode skin impedance monitoring for neurological disorders. In: IEEE 66th International Midwest Symposium on Circuits and Systems (MWSCAS) (2023)
13. Truong, N.D., et al.: Integer convolutional neural network for seizure detection. IEEE J. Emerg. Sel. Topics Circuits Syst. **8**, 849–857 (2018)
14. Usman, S.M., Usman, M., Fong, S.: Epileptic seizures prediction using machine learning methods. In: Computational and Mathematical Methods in Medicine (2017)
15. Kaleem, M., Gurve, D., Guergachi, A., Krishnan, S.: Patient-specific seizure detection in long-term EEG using signal derived empirical mode decomposition based dictionary approach. J. Neural Eng. (2018)
16. Solaija, M.S.J., Saleem, S., Khurshid, K., Hassan, S.A., Kamboh, A.M.: Dynamic mode decomposition based epileptic seizure detection from scalp EEG. IEEE Access **6**, 38683–38692 (2018)
17. Alotaiby, T.N., Alshebeili, S.A., Alotaibi, F.M., Alrshoud, S.R.: Epileptic seizure prediction using CSP and LDA for scalp EEG signals. Comput. Intell. Neurosci. (2017)
18. Cui, S., Duan, L., Qiao, Y., Xiao, Y.: Learning EEG synchronization patterns for epileptic seizure prediction using bag-of-wave features. J. Amb. Intell. Hum. Comput. 1–16 (2018)

19. Zhao, S., Yang, J., Xu, Y., Sawan, M.: Binary single-dimensional convolutional network for seizure prediction. In: 2020 IEEE International Symposium on Circuits and Systems (ISCAS), pp. 1–5 (2020)
20. Li, K.-C., Chiu, C.-T., Hsiao, S.-C.: Semantic segmentation via enhancing context information by fusing multiple high-level features. In: 2020 IEEE Workshop on Signal Processing Systems (SiPS), 2020, pp. 1–5 (2020)
21. Yang, X., Zhao, J., Sun, Q., Lu, J., Ma, X.: An effective dual self-attention residual network for seizure prediction. IEEE Trans. Neural Syst. Rehabil. Eng. **29**, 1604–1613 (2021)
22. Rasheed, K., Qadir, J., O'Brien, T.J., Kuhlmann, L., Razi, A.: A generative model to synthesize EEG data for epileptic seizure prediction. IEEE Trans. Neural Syst. Rehabil. Eng. **29**, 2322–2332 (2021)
23. Truong, N.D., et al.: Convolutional neural networks for seizure prediction using intracranial and scalp electroencephalogram. Neural Networks **105**, 104–111 (2018)
24. Zhang, X., Li, H.: Patient-specific seizure prediction from scalp EEG using vision transformer. In: 2022 IEEE 6th Information Technology and Mechatronics Engineering Conference (ITOEC), pp. 1663–1667 (2022)
25. Ryu, S., Joe, I.: A hybrid DenseNet-LSTM model for epileptic seizure prediction. Appl. Sci. **16**, 7661 (2021)
26. Liang, D., et al.: A novel consistency-based training strategy for seizure prediction. J. Neurosci. Methods **372**, 109557 (2022)
27. Dissanayake, T., Fernando, T., Denman, S., Sridharan, S., Fookes, C.: Deep learning for patient-independent epileptic seizure prediction using scalp EEG signals. IEEE Sens. J. **21**(7), 9377–9388 (2021)
28. Zhang, Q., Ding, J., Kong, W., Liu, Y., Wang, Q., Jiang, T.: Epilepsy prediction through optimized multidimensional sample entropy and Bi-LSTM. Biomed. Signal Process. Control **64**, 102293 (2021)
29. Zhang, Q., et. al.: Spatio-temporal-spectral hierarchical graph convolutional network with semisupervised active learning for patient-specific seizure prediction. IEEE Trans. Cybernet. (2021)
30. Sun, B., et al.: Seizure prediction in scalp EEG based channel attention dual-input convolutional neural network. Phys. A **584**, 126376 (2021)
31. Zhang, S., et al.: A lightweight solution to epileptic seizure prediction based on EEG synchronization measurement. J. Supercomput. **77**(4), 3914–3932 (2021)
32. Gao, Y., et al.: Pediatric seizure prediction in scalp EEG Using a multi-scale neural network with dilated convolutions. IEEE J. Transl. Eng. Health Med. **10**, 1–9 (2022). Art no. 4900209
33. Usman, S.M., Khalid, S., Bashir, Z.: Epileptic seizure prediction using scalp electroencephalogram signals. Biocybernet. Biomed. Eng. **41**(1), 211–220 (2021)
34. Halawa, R.I., Youssef, S.M., Elagamy, M.N.: An efficient hybrid model for patient-independent seizure prediction using deep learning. Appl. Sci. **12**(11), 5516 (2022)
35. Meng, Q., Catchpoole, D., Skillicom, D., Kennedy, P.J.: Relational autoencoder for feature extraction. In: International Joint Conference on Neural Networks (IJCNN) 2017, pp. 364–371 (2017)
36. Blagus, R., Lusa, L.: SMOTE for high-dimensional class-imbalanced data. BMC Bioinform. **14**(1), 1–16 (2013)
37. Ahmad, M.Z., Kamboh, A.M., Saleem, S., Khan, A.A.: Mallat's scattering transform based anomaly sensing for detection of seizures in scalp EEG. IEEE Access **5**, 16919–16929 (2017)
38. Hossain, M.S., Amin, S.U., Alsulaiman, M., Muhammad, G.: Applying deep learning for epilepsy seizure detection and brain mapping visualization. ACM Trans. Multimed. Comput. Commun. Appl. **15**, 1–17 (2019)
39. Boo, Y., Shin, S., Sung, W.: Quantized neural networks: characterization and holistic optimization. In: 2020 IEEE Workshop on Signal Processing Systems (SiPS), pp. 1–6 (2020)

40. Selvakumari, R.S., Mahalakshmi, M., Prashalee, P.: Patient-Specific Seizure Detection Method using Hybrid Classifier with Optimized Electrodes. J. Med. Syst. 43–121 (2019)
41. Tăuțan, A.M., Dogariu M., Ionescu, B.: Detection of epileptic seizures using unsupervised learning techniques for feature extraction. In: 41st International Conference of the IEEE Engineering in Medicine and Biology Society (EMBC), Berlin, pp. 2377–2381 (2019)
42. Alkanhal, I., Kumar, B.V.K.V., Savvides, M.: Automatic seizure detection via an optimized image-based deep feature learning. In: 17th IEEE International Conference on Machine Learning and Applications (ICMLA), Orlando, FL, pp. 536–540 (2018)
43. Yang, J.: Parameter selection of Gaussian kernel SVM based on local density of training set. Inverse Probl. Sci. Eng. **29**(4), 536–548 (2021)
44. Shoeb, A.H.: Application of machine learning to epileptic seizure onset detection and treatment. Ph.D. diss., Massachusetts Institute of Technology (2009)
45. Zhu, B., Farivar, M., Shoaran, M.: ResOT: resource-efficient oblique trees for neural signal classification. IEEE Trans. Biomed. Circuits Syst. **14**(4), 692–704 (2020)
46. Akbulut, Y., Sengur, A., Guo, Y., Smarandache, F.: NS-k-NN: neutrosophic set-based k-nearest neighbors classifier. Symmetry **9**(9), 179 (2017)

Topic Modelling and Interpretable Cost Estimation for Medical Insurance Fraud Detection

James Kemp[1]({{:}}), Christopher Barker[2], Norm Good[3], and Michael Bain[1]

[1] University of New South Wales, Sydney, NSW, Australia
`{james.kemp,m.bain}@unsw.edu.au`
[2] Australian Government Department of Health and Aged Care, Sydney, NSW, Australia
`chris.barker2@health.gov`
[3] Commonwealth Scientific and Industrial Research Organisation, Canberra, QLD, Australia
`norm.good@csiro.au`

Abstract. Medical insurance incurs significant costs and can be susceptible to fraud or waste. Machine learning approaches to automating fraud detection are becoming commonplace. Real-world pipelines including decision support systems for compliance activities on medical insurance claims may include requirements such human-interpretability and estimates of recoverable costs, to assist with prioritisation and investigation. We previously developed a framework for learning claim contexts and provider roles, incorporating domain knowledge through the insurance item ontology, and ranking providers for audit based on cost differences between similar providers. We extend this by comparing an interpretable pattern-identification cost estimator to the original scoring method and evaluating on a large real-world claims dataset. Compared to our previous cost estimator performance was similar, but with the advantage of immediately interpretable results. Results show incorporating context discovery and domain knowledge into fraud detection algorithms assists identification of comparable providers and generation of interpretable results for subject-matter experts in the decision-support process.

Keywords: Unsupervised machine learning · Data mining · Orthopedic procedures · National health insurance · Fraud

1 Introduction

The integrity of public service-providing organisations can be undermined by potentially illegal or profligate activity. An example is provision of government-subsidised healthcare, which in many countries is a significant proportion of the budget, and can be liable to waste or fraud [5, 14]. On one estimate individual healthcare organisations in OECD countries can be susceptible to fraud at the level of between 3% and 8% of

---

This research is supported by an Industry PhD scholarship which includes funding from the Commonwealth Scientific and Industrial Research Organisation, the Department of Health, Australian Government, and an Australian Government Research Training Program (RTP) scholarship.

overall expenditure [18]. In Australia, the federal government reimburses healthcare providers for services rendered under the Medicare Benefits Schedule (MBS), which categorises and itemises eligible hospital and medical service costs, while provision of medications is covered under the separate Pharmaceutical Benefits Scheme (PBS) [15]. The annual allocated budget amount in 2022–23 for total Australian Government expenditure on health is over $A 100 billion [30]. If the OECD estimates are applicable to Medicare Australia, significant taxpayer losses could be involved. Moreover, rates of detection of fraud and waste in healthcare in Australia have been estimated to be less than 1%, which is low compared to other countries [13].

Given the volume and variety of data that must be analysed at scale, machine learning is clearly a tool that may improve detection [14,16,27]. However, finding patterns suggestive of potential waste or fraud that can lead to significant cost recovery is typically a complex, time-consuming process of compliance checking led by human domain specialists into which machine learning methods must fit [14]. This leads to several challenges for machine learning.

Since instances of potentially suspicious behaviour must be reviewed by human experts in both medical specialities and compliance, obtaining labelled data is difficult. Even if this were possible, the small amount of non-compliant cases detected as a proportion of all claims would lead to highly unbalanced class ratios. Also, changes over time in regulation and provider claiming behaviour mean that historical data becomes rapidly "stale" and of limited use in training models. Applications of unsupervised learning to fraud detection problems have, therefore, usually been framed in terms of anomaly detection, using techniques such as clustering or outlier scoring [16]. However such methods can lack interpretability since they may not provide information on the patterns of activity on which outlier scores are based, and are typically limited in being able to incorporate information from relevant domain knowledge.

In previous work [21,23,24] we developed several models addressing requirements for real-world use of machine learning for anomaly detection in medical insurance claims. The requirements included: (1) use of unsupervised learning; (2) techniques generalisable to classes of problems within medical insurance claims; (3) interpretability of results; (4) automated discovery of similar claim contexts; and (5) estimation of potential cost recovery. These five requirements are grounded in the challenges inherent in the healthcare domain [22].

Each of our previous models addressing these requirements was validated by subject-matter experts at the Australian Government Department of Health and Aged Care, and shown to be useful for identifying providers at high-risk of non-compliance with the Medicare Benefits Schedule (MBS).

1.1 Research Goals

This paper is an extension of [21]. We substantially update the original work with clearer methodological descriptions, expand the requirements for the project, and add new research which develops the original work with three principal goals:

1. To detail the working of Graphical Association Analysis, which the model we are exploring can be built on.

2. To synthesise the interpretable end-results algorithm from our sequential pattern mining model [24] into the procedure model [21], thereby expanding the utility of the model by providing explicit identification of items which contribute to the cost ranking.
3. To highlight the benefits of modular model design, allowing flexibility in model construction [22].

We will address these goals in terms of the five requirements stated above.

Unsupervised Learning. Class labels for supervised learning can be costly to create due to the large numbers and variety of health insurance claims, and the expertise required to analyse them [16]. Moreover, health insurance claiming behaviour changes rapidly, as medical guidelines and health insurance policies are updated, and as abusers of the insurance systems adjust to compliance activities. This rapid concept drift means that class labels lose their utility [1]. Unsupervised learning methods for clustering and outlier detection are therefore preferable, as current behaviours can be learned directly from the data. However, studies directly comparing supervised and unsupervised methods have shown that further research is required on unsupervised learning in this domain [6,16].

Model Generality. Many published models are designed and tested on a single provider speciality or set of items, and may be ineffective when applied to other types of investigation, or where the data contains mixtures of specialist claims [7]. Constructing new models for each class of problem is time-consuming, so models with general applicability are desirable.

Human-Interpretable Results. Machine identification of potential non-compliance can be viewed as the first stage of a compliance process, which may result in audits or other compliance activities [29]. In a decision support system, interpretable models can improve trust in the results, expedite the subsequent stages (as the nature of the non-compliance can be more readily identified), and reduce potential for legal issues should recovery activities end in court. Few studies have addressed this concern, and many models lack clear human interpretation [8].

Recoverable Cost Estimation. Considerable variation in medical practice between providers is to be expected due to differing administration, patient demographics, and training. Anomalies due to this inherent variation are common, and are often of little interest to compliance analysts. Audits and other interventions can be costly for the department, and providers and industry bodies often push back on attempts to address problem claiming. Estimating the recoverable costs for non-compliant behaviour can help determine priority for investigators, and thresholds for segmentation can be applied at a desired return on investment, which is less arbitrary than for some methods [16,37].

Context Discovery. Investigating single-instance anomalous claims, or *point anomalies* [2], only highlights the variation in medical practice across patients, providers or administrative processes. *Contextually anomalous* providers can be found when they repeatedly behave differently from similar providers in similar situations [2,37]. Identifying similar providers in heterogeneous medical insurance data can be difficult. While providers in Australia have a registered speciality, their practice may change over time and the speciality they registered for may not reflect their abilities or the patients they see. Many items are ubiquitous, and have a high degree of overlap between specialities. In regional areas, where staff are not readily available, cross-training is common and service co-claims explicitly disallowed by the MBS may be permitted by Services Australia staff under these circumstances. Similar circumstances may legitimately generate very different claims, and vice-versa. The relationships between items which form the *context* in which they can and should occur, therefore, is determined by domain knowledge and cannot be discovered solely from data; an ideal model would incorporate this domain knowledge in a machine-friendly way.

2 Methods

2.1 Data

The Medicare Program in Australia provides reimbursement for medical services and hospital care for Australian residents and some visitors. Eligible services and reimbursement amounts are defined by the MBS as an ontology with a tree structure representing the relationship between items [3]. The tree comprises five levels: $Category \rightarrow Group \rightarrow Subgroup \rightarrow Subheading \rightarrow Item$ (with subgroup and subheading being optional). Reimbursement claims are recorded as rows in a tabular dataset, containing a claim for a single professional service performed according to the MBS, with information such as provider and patient identifiers, date of service, the item code (representing the service performed), and other relevant details. Conceptually, each row in the dataset can be considered a five-tuple $\langle D, I, A, V, F \rangle$, for $D \in Dates$, $I \in Item\ Codes$, $A \in Patients$, $V \in Providers$ and $F \in Fees$. Multiple services may be claimed on the same date, e.g., it may be appropriate for a consultation to occur before a surgery, both of which are separate items in the MBS. For this study, we used MBS claims data from 01-Oct-2019 to 30-Sep-2020.[1]

2.2 Data Extraction

To provide real-world relevance to the project and enable comparison with currently used approaches (see Sect. 2.9), a number of *target items* were chosen to match those of an existing investigation in progress at the DoH. The target items were all procedures related to either hand surgery (MBS Category 3: Therapeutic Procedures, Group T8: Surgical Operations, Subgroup 14: Hand Surgery), or orthopaedic surgery (MBS

---

[1] Owing to privacy concerns it will not be possible to release this dataset. Source code is available: https://github.com/jpkemp/anomaly_detection_framework.

Category 3: Therapeutic Procedures, Group T8: Surgical Operations, Subgroup 15: Orthopaedic).

From the claim dataset, a set of *patient events* was created. A patient event contains all claim rows for a single patient which shared the date of service for at least one claim from the defined categories of interest, i.e., all claims for a patient on the day of a claim for a target item for that patient. Specifically, for given date d, patient a and provider v, a patient event E is the set of all five-tuples $\langle D = d, I, A = a, V, F \rangle$ in the dataset.

Table 1 shows an example where patient events for two fictitious patients are identified for target items. In this example the first patient event for Patient 1 is identified due to the claim of a knee replacement procedure (item code 49518) on January 30. Three further items for Patient 1 claimed on the same date are also included in the patient event (note that two providers are involved). Patient 1 also has a second patient event based on the claim of a different target item, a shoulder replacement procedure (item code 48918) on August 1. On this second date a different patient event is also identified, a knee replacement for Patient 2, with three different providers included in this patient event.

Table 1. An example of claim rows (fictitious data) showing items claimed for two patients identified by target item (Knee or Shoulder replacement) and separated by date and patient ID to create three patient events involving four providers (see text for details) [21].

Patient ID	Provider ID	Item Code	Item Summary	Date
1	1	49518	Knee replacement	30-Jan
1	2	17610	Anaesthetic consultation	30-Jan
1	2	21402	Anaesthetic initiation	30-Jan
1	2	22031	Pain management	30-Jan
1	1	48918	Shoulder replacement	01-Aug
1	2	17610	Anaesthetic consultation	01-Aug
1	2	21622	Anaesthetic initiation	01-Aug
2	3	49518	Knee replacement	01-Aug
2	3	105	Professional attendance	01-Aug
2	2	17610	Anaesthetic consultation	01-Aug
2	2	21402	Anaesthetic initiation	01-Aug
2	4	51303	Surgical assistant	01-Aug

We define *episode pairs*, based on patient events, where each pair contains a *provider episode* and an *ontology episode*. A provider episode contains the list of items from a patient event claimed by a single provider. That is, for an event E, a provider episode e for a provider v is defined as:

$$e = \{r_2 | r \in E, r_4 = v\} \qquad (1)$$

where r_2 is the second element (containing the item code) and r_4 is the fourth element (containing the provider identifier) of the five-tuple r representing each claim row in E, as defined in Sect. 2.1.

For example, if three providers were involved in a patient event, the items from the patient event would be split into three separate provider episodes, each containing the list of items claimed by that provider. Table 2 shows the three provider episodes that would be generated from the patient event for Patient 2 in Table 1.

Table 2. Fictitious claim rows illustrating how claims in a patient event are separated by provider ID. Provider episodes are created from the items in the separated claim rows for each (Patient ID, Provider ID) pair on a given date of service [21].

Patient ID	Provider ID	Item Code	Item Summary	Date
2	3	49518	Knee replacement	01-Aug
2	3	105	Professional attendance	01-Aug
2	2	17610	Anaesthetic consultation	01-Aug
2	2	21402	Anaesthetic initiation	01-Aug
2	4	51303	Surgical assistant	01-Aug

An ontology episode contains a set of features denoting the *ontology location* of each item in the corresponding provider episode. For a given item, its ontology location is automatically derived by mapping each item code to a tuple containing its ancestors in the ontology tree, i.e., the item's Category, Group, Subgroup, and Subheading in the MBS ontology (see Fig. 1). Each tuple is converted to a single string, i.e., a feature, for

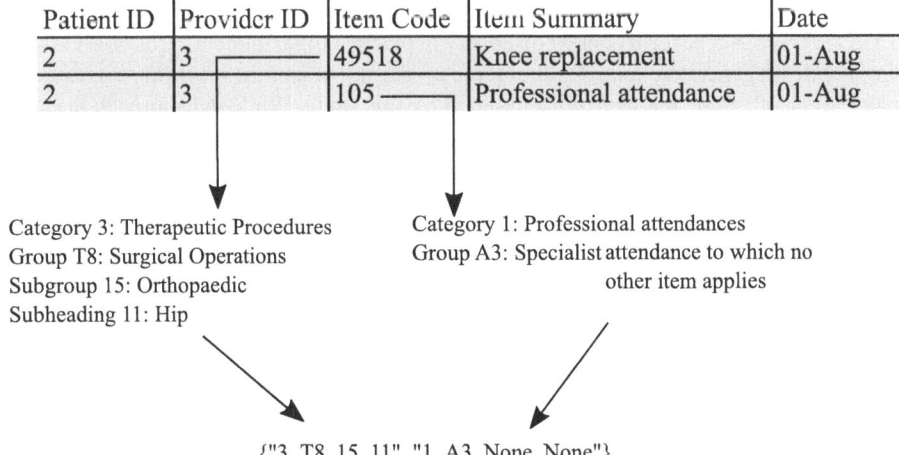

Fig. 1. Depiction of the items in a provider episode being mapped to their ontology locations in order to create an ontology episode [21].

the purposes of input to a learning algorithm to enable role modelling (see Sect. 2.3). This mapping reduced the 5953 individual item codes to 551 ontology locations [3]. Using the MBS ontology structure in this way creates a natural and interpretable prioritisation of relationships by innately identifying some close connections. In terms of feature construction, the ontology locations represent the least general generalisation of item codes with respect to the MBS ontology [19].

2.3 Role Modelling

Topic modelling is a form of unsupervised learning developed in text analysis to identify themes and their relationships within documents, which can then be used to classify documents according to those themes. Patient claims can be viewed as documents, and themes based on item relationships discovered using topic modelling. To give an initial context to the patient claims, the data was first grouped by the likely primary surgery. Episode pairs were assigned to a *subheading collection* by finding the ontology location of the highest-cost hand surgery or orthopaedic item within the parent patient event. The hand surgery group has no subheadings, and the orthopaedic group has 21 subheadings, resulting in 22 potential subheading collections. The *episode cost* for an episode pair was calculated by summing the schedule fees for the items in the provider episode. Several fee-based features are available in each claim row in the MBS. The schedule fee is the base fee rate for an item, before incentive payments or variable provider charges are applied. Variation in benefits paid to providers making the same claims can be attributed to government incentives with respect to location or other factors. Given that there is legitimate variation in fees, using other fee types such as the total benefit paid can lead to spurious results. The schedule fee is therefore the most comparable fee type for examining wasteful claims.

For each subheading collection, the associated episode pairs were passed to a *role modelling algorithm*. In [21], two algorithms were examined for the purpose of context discovery: Graphical Association Analysis (GAA) [23] and Latent Dirichlet Allocation (LDA) [9]. We use the term context discovery in place of topic modelling, as GAA is not a probabilistic generative model. Other topic modelling or context discovery algorithms may also be effective, but were not examined for this study. While the approach in each method is quite different, they can both be used to perform the same task, namely that of identifying typical roles of providers from the data. Essentially, typical roles within a surgery - e.g., surgeon, anaesthetist, assistant, etc. - were learned from the discovered relationships between the ontology locations contained in the ontology episodes.

2.4 Graphical Association Analysis

Association Analysis. For a given set of items (e.g., item codes from medical claims) and a set of transactions (each containing a subset of the items, representing one sample or instance), association analysis (AA) finds associations, in the form of rules, between items based on co-occurrence within transactions [32]. Association rules (ARs) have an antecedent and a consequent, meaning that if the antecedent is present in a transaction, it is anticipated the consequent will also be present. Antecedents and consequents may each contain multiple items ("itemsets"). Many algorithms for finding ARs exist, including exhaustive search, Apriori and FP-growth [32].

Reference and Provider Model Transaction Set. A provider episode is equivalent to an association analysis transaction. A transaction set T_s was constructed for each subheading collection s. More precisely, T_s is constructed as the set of n provider episodes e_i which are assigned to s, as follows:

$$T_s = \{e_1, e_2, ...e_n\} \; \forall e_i \text{ such that } (e_i, o_i) \in s, \; 1 \leq i \leq n. \tag{2}$$

where (e_i, o_i) represents the provider/ontology episode pair.

Unsupervised Learning of Graph Models. While items in transactions can be described in several ways, including common techniques such as one-hot encoding, graphs provide several benefits, including: ease of visualisation, maintaining item associations, and the ability to segment data by identifying the graph component to which items belong. As unsupervised learning is based on identifying subsets of related items in data, it can be viewed as a graph problem. That is, it can naturally be conceived of as a network of relationships between the items. Association analysis is applied using a probabilistic measure to identify edges between items which were then combined into graphs for cost analysis, provider ranking and visualization. Association rules provide a probabilistic definition of graph edges where distance metrics may be difficult to define [20]. To construct reference models of typical items claimed in transactions, a specialised form of AR mining was implemented to create directed graphs (digraphs) of item associations (for an example, see Fig. 2). As there are typically large numbers of rules discovered with AA, many of which may be irrelevant or spurious, interest measures are used to filter rules [32,34]. Two such measures were chosen for this study: support and conviction.

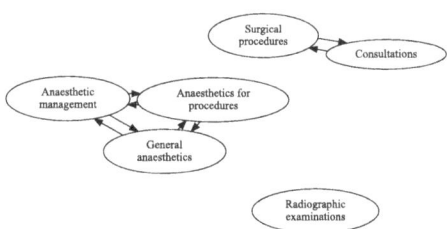

Fig. 2. Fictitious graph illustrating how GAA can learn provider roles. The 2-item component represents surgeon claims, the 3-item component represents anaesthetist claims, and the 1-item component represents radiologist claims [21].

Support is a measure of frequency, i.e., how often the itemset appears across all the transactions. It is commonly chosen because itemsets that rarely occur may occur only by chance. For a transaction set T, support σ for an itemset X is defined as:

$$\sigma(X) = \frac{|\{e \in T | X \subseteq e\}|}{|T|} \qquad (3)$$

Confidence c of an AR measures how frequently itemset Y co-occurs in transactions containing X, defined as:

$$c(X \to Y) = \frac{\sigma(X \cup Y)}{\sigma(X)} \qquad (4)$$

Conviction, which we denote as t, is an asymmetric measure (giving direction to the co-occurrence relationship) which determines whether there is a positive ($t > 1$), negative ($t < 1$), or independent ($t = 1$) association between antecedent and consequent itemsets — essentially, it is designed to discover likely implications between antecedent and consequent [11]. Conviction has been shown to be an effective predictive measure of interest for classification [4]. Support and confidence are used in determining conviction. Conviction t is defined as:

$$t(X \to Y) = \frac{1 - \sigma(Y)}{1 - c(X \to Y)} = \frac{1 - P(Y)}{1 - P(Y|X)} = \frac{P(\overline{Y})}{1 - P(Y|X)} = \frac{P(X)P(\overline{Y})}{P(X \cap \overline{Y})} \qquad (5)$$

where $\overline{Y}$ denotes the non-occurrence of itemset Y in transactions.

As an example, consider a dataset $\mathcal{D}$ of 1,000 transactions, 400 of which contain itemset X. Support $\sigma(X)$ in $\mathcal{D}$ is then 0.4. Now if 320 of those transactions containing X also contain itemset Y then $c(X \to Y) = 0.8$. That is, confidence is the conditional probability $P(Y|X)$ with respect to $\mathcal{D}$.

It might be thought that confidence can be used to detect any rule that can form an edge in the graph. However, it could happen that if both itemsets X and Y are probabilistically independent but occur very frequently a rule $X \to Y$ may have high confidence. In such a case, suppose $P(X) = P(Y) = 0.9$. We then have $c(X \to Y) = 0.9$, although the rule is spurious.

The problem is due to the fact that $P(Y)$ is not used in calculating confidence. Measures based on testing for the probabilistic independence of X and Y, such as "interest" [11], could be used, but they are symmetric, leading to the construction of an undirected graph. Several measures of interestingness, including conviction, are asymmetric in the sense of aligning with the dependence of consequent on antecedent in an AR [34]. Conviction, which was introduced and named in the context of association rule mining [34] is however essentially the same as an earlier measure from statistics [28]. Conviction has performed well and was also selected for this study [23]. Other interest measures may also perform well with AR learning for graphs; different measures of this type may be more or less suitable in different domains [34]. Note that conviction is defined to reach a maximum value of ∞ when the antecedent of an AR is a perfect predictor of the consequent (which is unlikely to occur on real data). In this study the conviction threshold was set to > 1 to capture only positive associations between antecedent and consequent.

To simplify the graph structure, both the antecedent and consequent within any AR were restricted to contain only a single item. ARs are discovered by evaluating support and conviction between each item pair (x, y) in the data. An AR $x \rightarrow y$ is selected if its support and conviction are higher than pre-specified thresholds. If a transaction contained only one item, a null item was temporarily added so that the AR mining algorithm can detect a single item as a typical transaction. A set of edges in the form of ordered pairs representing the antecedent and consequent, respectively, of each discovered AR is then created for each procedure subset in the dataset. The set of all items occurring as either antecedent or consequent of any discovered AR comprise the set of vertices. These sets of vertices and edges make up the digraphs, i.e., the graph models, which form the basis of this approach.

Reference Model Construction. Reference models describing typical claims made by providers for each of the three procedures were constructed from the respective transaction set T_s as described in Sect. 2.4. A reference model is a directed graph (digraph) relating items in the transaction set.

Support thresholds for AR mining were set to values between 0.01 and 0.08 in 0.01 increments for each reference model, for use in a sensitivity analysis. For the final reference models used to create results for validation, the support threshold was set to 0.05; this threshold has been previously validated for similar work [23]. Each vertex in the digraph represents an item code, each directed edge indicates an association, and each component in the graph is interpreted as the *role* of a class of providers in the procedure (e.g., surgeons, anaesthetists, etc.). Edge direction indicates the asymmetry provided by conviction.

Role Assignment. Because the ontology episodes are constructed on a per-patient, per-provider basis, and because different provider roles within a procedure utilise items from different ontology locations within the MBS, components of the graph indicate different provider roles within the procedure. Episode pairs were assigned to a role based on the closest matching component (i.e. the most matching ontology items). In learning the provider roles and contributing items within the procedure, GAA provides a context discovery method, with the advantage of easy visualisation using the graph structure which can help with human interpretability.

2.5 Latent Dirichlet Allocation

LDA is a Bayesian probabilistic graphical model which uses mixture models of items in collections over a set number of hidden topics [9]. Similarly to GAA, when applied to ontology episodes, modelled topics will find probabilities for ontology locations appearing in documents within that topic (see Table 3). Episode pairs were assigned to a role by finding the closest matching topic, i.e., the discovered topics define the provider roles. We arbitrarily assigned 5 topics, based on examination of the GAA results.

Table 3. Fictitious LDA topics illustrating how provider roles are learned. Topic 1 represents surgeon claims, topic 2 represents anaesthetist claims, and topic 3 represents radiologist claims [21].

Item	Topic 1	Topic 2	Topic 3
Surgical procedures	0.800	0.001	0.001
Consultations	0.150	0.001	0.050
Anaesthetics management	0.001	0.400	0.001
Anaesthetics for procedures	0.001	0.280	0.001
General anaesthetics	0.001	0.310	0.050
Radiographic examinations	0.047	0.048	0.897

2.6 Estimation of Provider Recoverable Costs: Weighted Median

For a given provider episode e, an episode cost f_e can be calculated as

$$f_e = \sum_{1}^{i} r_{i,5} \tag{6}$$

where $r_{i,5}$ denotes the element of the ith claim row tuple containing the cost for the claim.

The *expected cost* for a role within a context, regardless of the topic modelling algorithm, was calculated by taking the mean of the episode costs from the episode pairs associated with the role in a given context. That is, for the ith role, the expected cost

$$l_i = \frac{\sum_1^i f_i}{n_l} \tag{7}$$

where n_l is the number of episodes assigned to that role.

Each provider was assigned a *suspicion score*, representing the costs paid to the provider which might be recovered [21]. For the number of episodes pairs n_p associated with a given provider v, episode cost e_i for the ith episode and expected cost l_i for the role to which the relevant episode pair is assigned, the suspicion score s_v is

$$s_v = n_v \times \text{median}(\sum_{i=1}^{n} \max(e_i - l_i, 0)) \tag{8}$$

In this calculation, the median is used as it represents typical provider behaviour by ignoring outlying or extraordinary episodes, and is then weighted by the episode count for the provider. Episodes where the provider charges less than the expected l_i are ignored. Providers were then ranked by their suspicion score, with higher suspicion scores indicating possible repeated, expensive, and unusual activity. This score is designed to overcome the limitations of a method we used previously which focused solely on *items*, which does not adequately represent potential recoverable costs.

2.7 Alternate Cost Estimation: Itemised Cost

Each item claimed can be considered to have a distribution of claim rates across the providers within an ontology location and role, where the claim rate is the proportion of relevant provider episodes for a given provider in which the item is claimed. Co-occurrence of items, (i.e., where two items are claimed together) similarly have a distribution of claim rates.

We used the extreme outlier formula [35] to define a threshold for unusual providers for a given item being claimed, or pair of items co-claimed. That is, if a providers claim rate for an item or item pair exceeded the threshold

$$thresh_P = Q3 + 3 \times IQR \qquad (9)$$

where Q3 is the third quartile and IQR is the inter-quartile range, the provider was considered an unusual claimant of that item or item pair (we denote the item or item pair as a *pattern*). Providers with fewer than three episode pairs in a subheading collection were excluded from the distribution calculations, as their claim rates could not represent their typical behaviour and would be necessarily high.

With the idea that providers might be considered unusual for a given pattern, we can consider whether, with the claim rate for the pattern, they might be considered a normal claimant of a similar pattern. A similar pattern is one which contains one item from the unusual pattern, and either no other items (an extra item may have been claimed), or an item from the same ontology location as the other item in the given pattern (i.e., a similar item has been substituted in the providers claims, potentially indicating upcoding). If a provider is a normal claimant of a similar pattern, but unusual for the given pattern, we can say that the extra or substituted item is the unusual item in the claim, and we can recover the costs of the extra item, or the difference between the cost of the similar item and the claimed item in the case of a substitution. As multiple patterns can impact the same item, an item cost was only included once per episode regardless of how many relevant patterns it appeared in. These costs were summed to create the suspicion score for the provider. This method has an advantage over the weighted median scoring as it is explicit; the reasons for the high score can be traced directly to the unusual items.

2.8 Process Summary

The modelling and ranking process is summarised as follows:

1. Identify context
   (a) Identify the ontology location of the patient's primary surgery (e.g., knee, hip, shoulder)
   (b) Identify the provider's role within the patient event (e.g., surgeon, anaesthetist, assistant)
2. Calculate the typical fee for each role in each subheading collection
3. Calculate the suspicion score for each provider
   – *Either*
      (a) Calculate the differences between the episode cost and the typical cost of the assigned role for each episode pair

(b) Take the median difference for the episode pairs for each provider and weight by their total number of claims
- *Or*
  (a) Determine item claims/co-claims for which a provider's claim rate is unusual
  (b) Determine which items are causing the claim rate to be unusual
  (c) Sum the costs of the provider's unusual items
4. Rank providers by the suspicion score

2.9 Validation

Due to the volume of data both as input and output to these methods, validating the results is difficult. In order to determine whether the method is producing useful results, known anomalous providers as well as high-scoring, previously unknown providers were examined.

LDA Repeatability. As LDA is a stochastic method, the topics produced vary run to run, resulting in different episode role assignments. To reduce the effect of the variation, the LDA method was run multiple times, and the mean suspicion scores were used to determine the final rank. Two-way mixed effects intra-class correlation coefficients for both single fixed and average fixed raters (ICC3 and ICC3k) were used to measure the variation in the scores across the LDA runs, treating the providers as raters [25]. ICC3 measures within-rater reliability of a fixed group of raters over multiple ratings, whereas ICC3k measures mean rating score from a fixed group of raters over multiple ratings. In this way we can infer LDA consistency from the within-rater reliability of the provider scores produced across the runs. The ICCs were tested on log-transformed data, used to produce a normal distribution from the raw scores which were highly right-tailed. Descriptive statistics were done on the largest change in score for all providers as a proportion of the total schedule fees for their claims, i.e.

$$\text{changes} = \frac{\max(s_{i,v}) - \min(s_{i,v))}}{\text{total\_fees}(v)} \forall v \qquad (10)$$

where $s_{i,v}$ is the score for a given provider v in a single test run i, and total_fees is the sum of the provider's fees across all their episodes [21].

Rank-biased overlap (RBO) was used to measure the differences in the rankings across the LDA runs, as changes in the scores will affect the ranking. RBO is a metric for determining rank-ordered list overlap which has several advantages over similar metrics, including being symmetric, top-weighted, and not tail-dominated, which are consistent with the requirements for ranking in this study [36]. RBO was applied to all pairwise combination of ranks from the 10 runs. RBO was also used to compare the rankings of the top 100 providers from the LDA and GAA methods. A weight parameter of 0.99 was used with RBO to give 85% of the weight to the top 100 providers.

Comparison of Provider Ranking to Existing Information. Provider IDs were obtained for 100 surgical providers recently flagged as anomalous by the Compliance Analytics team at the DoH. These providers made claims from across the orthopaedic and hand-surgery MBS items, over the same time period as the data we used. They were identified using a variety of statistical analyses focusing on item claim and co-claim counts. We will refer to these 100 providers as the *anomalous set*, u. Let R denote the ordered set of the ranking of provider identifiers from either the GAA or LDA methods. The overlap between u and R was determined at 100 depths d_i, given by

$$d_i = \lfloor \frac{n \times i}{100} \rceil$$

where n is the number of providers in R, i is an integer in [1..100], and d_i is rounded to the nearest integer. The overlap o at a depth d_i is then

$$o_{d_i} = |u \cap \{v_1, v_2, ...v_{d_i} | v \in R\}| \qquad (11)$$

As well as the depths described above, the number of overlapping providers in the top 100 was calculated. This analysis indicated whether the ranking provided by our method is able to pick up known anomalies.

In-Depth Examination of Previously Unidentified Cases. High-scoring providers in our ranking who did not appear in the anomalous set were examined against their peers with methods currently in use at the DoH. As the method incorporates cost into the ranking, it is possible that the high-ranking providers typically handled more complex patient cases. The DoH assigns an in-house provider speciality label (PSL) to its providers based on the provider's registered specialty and their item claims over a quarter. We obtained the PSL for the top 20 providers in the GAA rankings which were not in the anomalous set; we will refer to these providers as the *high-scoring set*. Counts of item claims and co-claims were compiled from the provider episodes for all providers in each PSL, where provider episodes existed in the extracted patient events (i.e., the providers had claims in the extracted data from Sect. 2.2). For each of the high-scoring set providers, the number of claims and percentile of claims for each item and item co-claim was examined by hand to determine whether the provider was making unusual claims.

Outlying item counts for items claimed by at least 10 providers were also flagged using an adjusted boxplot outlier formula. By inspection, many of the items had a right-tailed, zero-inflated Poisson distribution, indicating a high proportion of providers did not claim given items at all. Typical outlier detection methods may not work well in this case as the distribution is both skewed and zero-inflated [33]. The outlier cutoff c was therefore calculated only on the positive-valued data, using the following formula to account for skew [33,38]:

$$c = Q_3 + 1.5 \times IQR \times e^{3MC}, \qquad (12)$$

where MC is the medcouple. The medcouple measures univariate distribution skewness, reducing the impact of outliers compared to the classical skewness coefficient [12].

This analysis indicated whether the previously unidentified providers were making unusual claims or merely expensive ones.

Suspicion Score Comparison. Since the study on which this extension paper is based was conducted, research funding has ended and the project has been taken up by other DoH staff. Research access is consequently more limited, and some resources (including the anomalous set and expert staff) were no longer available to the authors. Direct comparison of the alternate suspicion score to the results above has not been possible at time of submission, nor has access to the provider information required to perform manual analysis.

Tests were conducted between the two suspicion scores using the data specified, with GAA as the role modelling algorithm. Three methods were used to assess the performance of the alternate suspicion score. The RBO was calculated between the rankings from the weighted median metric and the alternate metric. Providers making claims at outlying rates were identified algorithmically as per Sect. 2.9, but applied to the top 20, 50, and 100 providers in the ranking regardless of whether they were in the anomalous set or not. In the initial study, we noted that the skew-adjusted outlier formula is not always calculable, and that it often resulted in conservative estimates [21]. The extreme outlier formula was, therefore, also used to evaluate the outliers. It was applied both the raw claim distributions, and to distributions normalised using the Box-Cox transformation [10].

2.10 Results

The extracted data comprised 1,918,643 claim rows from 31,306 providers covering 331,323 patient events. For the LDA runs, ICC3 on the log-transformed provider scores was 0.035 whereas ICC3k was > 0.99. This shows low consistency within the provider scores across the LDA runs, but good consistency in the mean scores. As a proportion of total costs, the median change was 0.12, the mean change was 0.15, and the maximum change was 0.97 indicating that most provider scores changed by only a small amount across the LDA runs, and only a small number of providers changed by a large amount. This is due to the episode assignment to roles changing as the topics change. Providers with many episodes which border on two different roles will have large changes in score as the role cost to which their episodes are compared changes. For example, if a provider typically claims episodes which contain both surgical and anaesthetic items (an uncommon edge case), as the topic weightings change the bulk of their episodes might be assigned to the topic representing the surgeon role, or the topic representing the anaesthetist role. As surgical procedure items tend to be relatively expensive, the episode costs may be close to the mean if they are assigned to the surgical role, but much higher than the mean if they are assigned to the anaesthetist role. This provider could then have either a low score or a high score, depending on the learned topics.

The RBO between the rankings from the LDA runs ranged from 0.51 to 0.86, with a mean of 0.74. This shows that the provider ranks can vary due to the stochastic nature of LDA, but in spite of the variation of the within-provider scores, a general agreement exists between the rankings. The RBO between the ranking from the GAA method and the combined ranking from the LDA method was 0.81, also showing agreement.

Known Anomalous Providers. Plots of the ranking overlap with the anomalous set are shown in Figs. 3 and 4 for the GAA and LDA methods respectively[2]. Of the 100 top-scoring providers from the GAA ranking, 28 were part of the anomalous set, and in the LDA results 33 of the top 100 were from the anomalous set. Most of the anomalous set providers ranked within the top 10% with both methods. The LDA method produced a steeper curve, ranking more of the anomalous higher than the GAA method. In both methods some of the anomalous providers ranked low, with a score of 0. From the plots, it can clearly be seen that the providers who have ranked highly are those with both more episodes and a higher cost per episode. This is in line with the objective of ranking providers based on potential return on investment, rather than solely on anomalous behaviour.

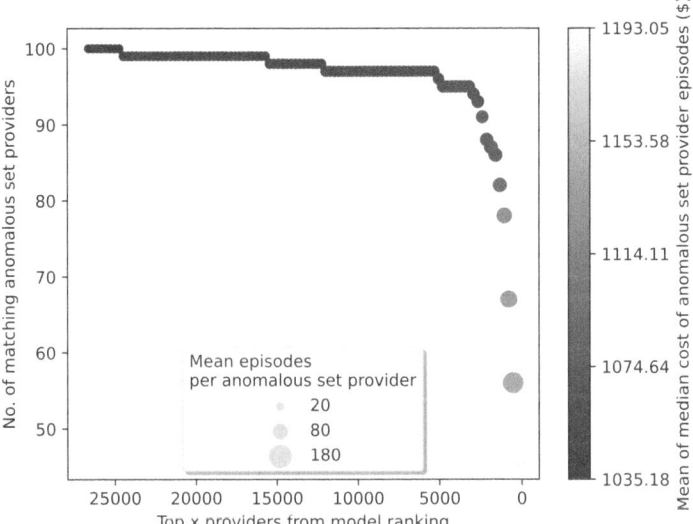

Fig. 3. GAA provider rankings showing the overlap with the anomalous set, with each circle representing 100%, 99%, 98%, and so on of the assessed providers. The anomalous set providers ranked more highly by the GAA method have more, and more expensive, episodes than the other anomalous set providers as indicated by the larger, lighter coloured circles as lower-ranked providers drop out of the cumulative analysis [21].

High-Scoring Providers. For privacy reasons we will only discuss the results in general terms – the points noted will also apply to other similar providers. The high-scoring sets included cardio-thoracic surgeons, general surgeons, orthopaedic surgeons, plastic and reconstructive surgeons, and anaesthetists. Seventeen providers overlapped in

---

[2] Note the number of providers in the GAA and LDA results is different due to GAA assigning some providers to no role, which was not assessed. The number of providers in each interval is therefore also different.

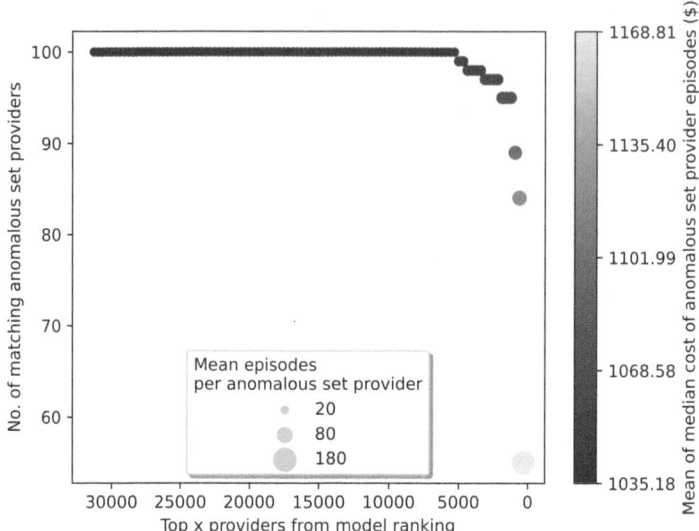

Fig. 4. LDA provider ranking overlap with the anomalous set at even intervals. The plot is constructed as per Fig. 3 [21].

the GAA and LDA high-scoring sets, totalling twenty-three providers examined. The results are summarised in Table 4

Two of the providers displayed behaviour that had previously been investigated; the quantity and type of items they claimed are common in a particular sub-speciality, and are unlikely to be an abuse of the system. Had this previous investigation not occurred, these surgeons would have been highlighted for further investigation. Four of the identified providers, whilst high-volume claimants of some items, were either claiming similar volumes to their near-peers, or were not engaging in potential upcoding or unusual co-claiming behavior. For a conservative estimate the claiming patterns for these providers are considered genuine.

The providers we designated unusual were in the top percentiles of claimants in their PSL for co-claimed items or items indicating potential upcoding or unbundling, with a large increase in number of claims from the percentiles below. Upcoding occurs when a similar, higher value claim is made in place of another service [14]. Upcoding patterns can also potentially indicate claims from senior consulting physicians who only take complex patients, however it is not possible to assess the difference from the claims data alone, and further investigation would be required. Unbundling occurs when multiple codes are billed in place of a cheaper 'bundled' item which is intended to cover the collection of services, and is a common target for recovery [14].

Similar numbers of providers were detected by the adjusted outlier detection formula as by hand. However, we found outlier detection on positive-valued data is quite conservative and not always appropriate. For example, one provider had several hundred claims of an item. The value at the 99th percentile (including 0-valued data) was

Table 4. High-scoring set providers confirmed as unusual [21].

Method	By hand	By formula	Assessed
GAA only	3	3	3
LDA only	2	3	3
Both	12 (14)	11	17
Total	17 (19)	17	23

around 16, but the provider was not flagged as an outlier. With most providers within a PSL not claiming that item, such a high volume of claims was considered of interest.

Cost Estimates. The RBO between the suspicion scores calculated from the weighted median and the itemised cost was 0.52, indicating that investigative priority might change considerably depending on the metric. The distribution of the both scores was remarkably right-tailed distributions, indicating that most providers have low potential recoverable costs relative to the outlying providers. That is, most providers were performing similarly within their roles and contexts, but some providers were notably different. The estimated recoverable costs were approximately one order of magnitude higher with the itemised cost than the weighted median, with means of approximately $A 14,000 and $A 1,400, and maximums of approximately $A 3 million and $A 450,000, respectively. Table 5 shows the number of outliers at several rank depths, as a proxy for accuracy. While the RBO indicates the rank ordering changed, both scoring methods identified similar numbers of providers who would be considered outliers from their peers according to the DoH.

Two points were noted by the analyst liaising with us regarding the alternate suspicion score. Firstly, for some providers and two-item patterns, no similar patterns were found despite the existence of potential candidates. This was due to the provider's claiming at an outlying rate even for the more common, shorter patterns. That is, the provider was found to be unusual with all similar patterns. We had not seen this occur in the oncology work on which the itemised score was based; among the high-scoring providers, similar patterns were always found for patterns containing more than one item. Secondly, some items were not assigned to an ontology location as they were not

Table 5. Providers making at least one item claim or co-claim in outlying rates.

Metric	Rank depth	Skew-adjusted	Normalised	Extreme
Itemised cost	20	15 (75%)	19 (95%)	18 (90%)
Weighted median	20	16 (80%)	20 (100%)	19 (95%)
Itemised cost	50	45 (90%)	49 (98%)	48 (96%)
Weighted median	50	43 (86%)	50 (100%)	48 (96%)
Itemised cost	100	92 (92%)	99 (99%)	95 (95%)
Weighted median	100	85 (85%)	100 (100%)	96 (96%)

contained in the version of the MBS we used for item lookup. That is, the item definitions changed over the course of the year of data we examined. Concept drift on item definitions can affect what is considered similar if ontology location changes or if items are changed or removed, leading to potentially incorrect similar patterns being discovered. This did not appear to impact the high-scoring providers in this study, but is worth noting. Item cost changes may also impact the outcome of future work.

3 Discussion

Data mining and statistical learning has a history of use in aiding decision-making [16,31]. By using topic modelling and incorporating domain knowledge encoded in the claim ontology structure, we are able to automatically group procedures and provider roles within those procedures, satisfying the requirement of context discovery. The cost estimation scores we demonstrate allow potential return to be estimated in an interpretable manner, and ranking providers by the magnitude of the difference to their peers is useful to decision makers in prioritising cases for action. Modularity of the design enables easily changing aspects of the pipeline, such as the topic modelling algorithm or the cost metric. The results showed that the method was able to detect both previously identified and novel patterns of potential fraud and waste. This method is therefore suitable as a decision-support tool for prioritisation of potential cases for audit, and for identifying patterns that can be encoded in other decision-support tools and used for identifying groups of providers exhibiting similar behaviour.

3.1 Challenges

Due to the heterogeneous nature of medical claims, not all providers in the anomalous set are engaging in fraudulent or wasteful behaviour. From the claims data alone it is very difficult to determine a genuine expert in a particularly complex or specialised procedure from one partaking in upcoding malpractice. Some providers perform services which border two different roles in a procedure, and depending on the role to which they are allocated, they might appear normal or expensive. This was highlighted by the high change in costs for some providers over repeated LDA runs. Any clustering approach will have the same problem on data with a high degree of overlap; some misclassification is inevitable, and no one tool is likely to be able to capture all fraudulent or wasteful practices [26]. It may be possible to assign multiple roles to an episode based on probabilities or perhaps Bayesian priors, however the method would need to be significantly extended to account for multiple potential scores. We consider some false-positives acceptable in a first stage decision-support tool, as the behaviours can then be identified, investigated, and assessed appropriately. Later-stage tools could incorporate known non-abuse patterns as a filter, or the knowledge could be fed back into the ontology structure to help group the providers more appropriately. Generally, the frequency of the patterns identified here were shown to be anomalous compared with the peer groups, as well as being expensive behaviours.

3.2 Topic Modelling

Both topic modelling methods discovered unusually costly providers with both known and unknown patterns of anomalous behaviour. There are advantages and disadvantages to each.

GAA offers the ability to drop episodes which do not fit the topics - classing them as not belonging to a role, which are not assessed - whereas LDA provides the most likely result. This classification could be useful as part of a decision-support suite, where episodes outside the typical part of a procedure could be sent to a different tool for further analysis. A threshold for similarity could be set to provide the same behaviour for LDA if required. The best approach may vary depending on the claims involved.

The GAA method is able to learn the number of roles, whereas LDA requires it to be specified beforehand. In this case the number set was based on visual examination of the GAA modelled roles. The best number of roles may not be fixed. In both cases, roles would need expert examination for suitability in a decision-support system; if the typical claims modelled by the topic-modelling algorithm did not make sense to subject-matter experts, the results of the ranking may not be appropriate.

3.3 Recoverable Cost Estimates

Some providers engaging in known anomalous behaviour were ranked very low by the weighted median scoring. Those providers were involved in cheaper procedures; while they exhibited some unbundling behaviour, their total costs were lower than their peers. Moreover, they were generally involved in fewer procedures than their peers. The providers who ranked highly were those involved in more, and more expensive, procedures. This is in accordance with the design goal of ranking by potential for return. Finer granularity in the MBS ontology could help better group the procedures so that complex, expensive procedures are not compared with simple ones.

The itemised cost scores tended to be much larger than the weighted median scores, and are potentially overestimates if specialist behaviour which is of little interest to auditors, but rarely performed, is being identified. Conversely, the weighted median score may be underestimating the recoverable costs, as it is our observation that providers in this domain who engage in potentially fraudulent behaviour will repeat the claims frequently. At this time, we are unable to determine which scoring method is more accurate, due to time and resource constraints on the experts required to validate the results. Regardless of the scoring, the itemised cost method has the benefit of being more explicitly interpretable by subject-matter experts, reducing the workload required to identify the reasons a provider is exhibiting unusual behaviour.

3.4 Model Limitations

The model design is based on two assumptions which warrant examination. The first assumption is that providers working within a similar area - i.e. a subheading collection - will see a similar distribution of patients and behave in a comparable manner. That is, it is assumed each provider will claim a similarly costed range of items within the subheading collection. In practice, distributions vary in part due to specialisation and seniority of the providers, meaning that the comparison between providers is not completely like-to-like. Junior practitioners will typically perform a far greater number of simple procedures, while senior practitioners and specialists will be involved in higher numbers of complex procedures, which would be more expensive.

The second assumption is that the ontology structure is consistent, i.e., that items within a subheading are equally related to each other and equally distant from items in a different subheading. Similarly, subheadings within a subgroup are assumed to be equally similar to each other, and equally distant from subheadings in a different subgroup. In practice, however, items do not function equivalently, and the structure of the ontology is not formulated for this purpose. However, it provides a simple and effective way of incorporating domain knowledge. These problems are inherent to data with a high degree of overlap, and are difficult to overcome.

3.5 Study Limitations

Validation of the models was necessarily limited through lack of availability of subject-matter experts able to review the results. Two fields of knowledge are required for these experts: specialist medical knowledge of the procedures, and knowledge of the legislation and policies that drives further action in recovering potentially fraudulent and wasteful claims. Few such people are employed by the DoH, and none were available for in-depth analysis, though they did provide assistance with our questions. The process for recovery is lengthy, and results based on outcomes of that process are also impractical to obtain at this stage. Review by data analysts at the DoH was considered to be adequate as the intent of the method is for a decision-support tool, and the data analysts would be the end-users, however a more thorough review would be beneficial. Use of the PSL for comparison purposes is not ideal, as it is known to be an imperfect tool for grouping similar providers. However, it is the tool that is currently in use, and as with all clustering problems there are multiple possible solutions each with advantages and disadvantages dependent on the use-case [17].

3.6 Future Work

Additional validation, such as ablation studies or further examination of the rankings and provider roles, including true negatives and mis-classified providers, may help improve the approach. However, due to resource constraints this was not possible for this study.

Further research could focus on better segregating similar providers. There are at least two ways this could be done. One option would be to make use of the cost distribution. Instead of using the median, it may be possible to examine distance from cost peaks. That may allow for different sub-specialties/seniority of providers working on a similar subheading collection. However, it may also lead to more blurring as low-scoring providers working similarly to providers from an expensive peak overlap with high-scoring providers working similarly to providers working from a cheaper peak. Weakly-supervised or seeded LDA would enable expert opinion to be included. Better incorporating domain knowledge into the ontology structure or the model would facilitate better results.

4 Conclusion

We present a modular model which meets the five requirements of unsupervised learning, generalisable techniques, interpretable results, automated context discovery, and estimation of potential cost recovery. The results show the utility of the model and highlight the challenges underlying this domain. With the extension of the alternate cost estimation, we improve on the interpretability of the model while maintaining performance.

Acknowledgements. This research is supported by an Industry PhD scholarship which includes funding from the Commonwealth Scientific and Industrial Research Organisation, the Department of Health, Australian Government, and an Australian Government Research Training Program (RTP) scholarship. Thanks to Dr. Joshua Myers at the DoH for assistance with creating the new material.

References

1. Abdallah, A., Maarof, M.A., Zainal, A.: Fraud detection system: a survey. J. Netw. Comput. Appl. **68**, 90–113 (2016). https://doi.org/10.1016/j.jnca.2016.04.007. http://www.sciencedirect.com/science/article/pii/S1084804516300571
2. Ariyaluran Habeeb, R.A., Nasaruddin, F., Gani, A., Targio Hashem, I.A., Ahmed, E., Imran, M.: Real-time big data processing for anomaly detection: a survey. Int. J. Inf. Manag. (2018). https://doi.org/10.1016/j.ijinfomgt.2018.08.006. http://www.sciencedirect.com/science/article/pii/S0268401218301658
3. Australian Government Department of Health: Medicare benefits schedule (2019)
4. Azevedo, P.J., Jorge, A.M.: Comparing rule measures for predictive association rules. In: Kok, J.N., Koronacki, J., Mantaras, R.L., Matwin, S., Mladenič, D., Skowron, A. (eds.) ECML 2007. LNCS (LNAI), vol. 4701, pp. 510–517. Springer, Heidelberg (2007). https://doi.org/10.1007/978-3-540-74958-5_47
5. Badgery-Parker, T., et al.: Low-value care in Australian public hospitals: prevalence and trends over time. BMJ Qual. Saf. **28**(3), 205 (2019). https://doi.org/10.1136/bmjqs-2018-008338. http://qualitysafety.bmj.com/content/28/3/205.abstract
6. Bauder, R., Khoshgoftaar, T.: Medicare fraud detection using machine learning methods. In: 2017 16th IEEE International Conference on Machine Learning and Applications (ICMLA), 18–21 December 2017, pp. 858–65. IEEE Computer Society (2017). https://doi.org/10.1109/ICMLA.2017.00-48
7. Bauder, R., Khoshgoftaar, T., Richter, A., Herland, M.: Predicting medical provider specialties to detect anomalous insurance claims. In: 2016 IEEE 28th International Conference on Tools with Artificial Intelligence (ICTAI), 6–8 November 2016, pp. 784–90. 2016 IEEE 28th International Conference on Tools with Artificial Intelligence (ICTAI). IEEE Computer Society (2017). https://doi.org/10.1109/ICTAI.2016.0123
8. Bauder, R.A., Khoshgoftaar, T.M.: The effects of varying class distribution on learner behavior for Medicare fraud detection with imbalanced big data. Health Inf. Sci. Syst. **6**(1), 9 (2018). https://doi.org/10.1007/s13755-018-0051-3
9. Blei, D.M., Ng, A.Y., Jordan, M.I.: Latent dirichlet allocation. J. Mach. Learn. Res. **3**, 993–1022 (2003)
10. Box, G.E., Cox, D.R.: An analysis of transformations. J. Roy. Stat. Soc. Ser. B (Methodol.) **26**(2), 211–243 (1964)

11. Brin, S., Motwani, R., Ullman, J.D., Tsur, S.: Dynamic itemset counting and implication rules for market basket data. In: Proceedings of the 1997 ACM SIGMOD International Conference on Management of Data - SIGMOD 1997, vol. 26, pp. 255—264. ACM Press (1997). https://doi.org/10.1145/253260.253325
12. Brys, G., Hubert, M., Struyf, A.: A robust measure of skewness. J. Comput. Graph. Stat. **13**(4), 996–1017 (2004). https://doi.org/10.1198/106186004X12632
13. Community Affairs Legislation Committee: Senate estimates Thursday 26 October (2017)
14. Couffinhal, A., Frankowski, A.: Wasting with intention: fraud, abuse, corruption and other integrity violations in the health sector, pp. 265–301. OECD Publishing (2017). https://doi.org/10.1787/9789264266414-10-en
15. Dixit, S.K., Sambasivan, M.: A review of the Australian healthcare system: a policy perspective. SAGE Open Med. **6** (2018). https://doi.org/10.1177/2050312118769211. https://www.ncbi.nlm.nih.gov/pubmed/29686869
16. Ekin, T., Ieva, F., Ruggeri, F., Soyer, R.: Statistical medical fraud assessment: exposition to an emerging field. Int. Stat. Rev. **86**(3), 379–402 (2018). https://doi.org/10.1111/insr.12269. https://www.scopus.com/inward/record.uri?eid=2-s2.0-85046363159&doi=10.1111%2finsr.12269&partnerID=40&md5=72f03c522aa78b41b2e0721b32f541fc
17. Estivill-Castro, V.: Why so many clustering algorithms: a position paper. SIGKDD Explor. Newsl. **4**(1), 65–75 (2002). https://doi.org/10.1145/568574.568575
18. Gee, J., Button, M.: The financial cost of healthcare fraud. Technical report, PKF Littlejohn LLP and University of Portsmouth (2015). https://pure.port.ac.uk/ws/portalfiles/portal/17778636/The_Financial_Cost_of_Healthcare_Fraud_Report_2015.pdf
19. Han, J., Kamber, M., Pei, J.: Data Mining: Concepts and Techniques. Morgan Kaufmann, Burlington (2011)
20. Huang, Z., Li, J., Su, H., Watts, G.S., Chen, H.: Large-scale regulatory network analysis from microarray data: modified Bayesian network learning and association rule mining. Decis. Support Syst. **43**(4), 1207–1225 (2007). https://doi.org/10.1016/j.dss.2006.02.002. https://www.sciencedirect.com/science/article/pii/S0167923606000248
21. Kemp, J., Barker, C., Good, N., Bain, M.: Context discovery and cost prediction for detection of anomalous medical claims, with ontology structure providing domain knowledge. In: Proceedings of the 16th International Joint Conference on Biomedical Engineering Systems and Technologies - Volume 5: HEALTHINF, pp. 29–40. SCITEPRESS, California, USA (2023)
22. Kemp, J., Barker, C., Good, N., Bain, M.: Developing an anomaly detection framework for Medicare claims. In: ACSW 2023: Australasian Computer Science Week 2023, pp. 234–237. Association for Computing Machinery, New York (2023)
23. Kemp, J., Barker, C., Good, N., Bain, M.: Graphical association analysis for identifying variation in provider claims for joint replacement surgery. In: Proceedings of the 19th World Congress on Medical and Health Informatics. IOS Press, Amsterdam, Holland (2023, accepted for publication)
24. Kemp, J., Barker, C., Good, N., Bain, M.: Sequential pattern detection for identifying courses of treatment and anomalous claim behaviour in medical insurance. In: 2022 IEEE International Conference on Bioinformatics and Biomedicine (BIBM), pp. 3039–3046 (2022). https://doi.org/10.1109/BIBM55620.2022.9995541
25. Koo, T., Li, M.: A guideline of selecting and reporting intraclass correlation coefficients for reliability research. J. Chiropractic Med. **15** (2016). https://doi.org/10.1016/j.jcm.2016.02.012
26. Kose, I., Gokturk, M., Kilic, K.: An interactive machine-learning-based electronic fraud and abuse detection system in healthcare insurance. Appl. Soft Comput. **36**, 283–299 (2015). https://doi.org/10.1016/j.asoc.2015.07.018. http://www.sciencedirect.com/science/article/pii/S1568494615004585

27. Krumholz, H.M.: Big data and new knowledge in medicine: the thinking, training, and tools needed for a learning health system. Health Aff. **33**(7), 1163–70 (2014). https://doi.org/10.1377/hlthaff.2014.0053
28. Loevinger, J.: A systematic approach to the construction and evaluation of tests of ability. Psychol. Monogr. **61**(4), 1–49 (1947). https://doi.org/10.1037/h0093565
29. Massi, M.C., Ieva, F., Lettieri, E.: Data mining application to healthcare fraud detection: a two-step unsupervised clustering method for outlier detection with administrative databases. BMC Med. Inform. Decis. Mak. **20**(1), 160 (2020). https://doi.org/10.1186/s12911-020-01143-9
30. Parliament of Australia: Health overview (2023). https://www.aph.gov.au/About_Parliament/Parliamentary_departments/Parliamentary_Library/pubs/rp/BudgetReview202223/HealthOverview
31. Sivarajah, U., Kamal, M.M., Irani, Z., Weerakkody, V.: Critical analysis of big data challenges and analytical methods. J. Bus. Res. **70**, 263–286 (2017). https://doi.org/10.1016/j.jbusres.2016.08.001. http://www.sciencedirect.com/science/article/pii/S014829631630488X
32. Tan, P.N.: Introduction to Data Mining, 2nd edn. Pearson Education Inc., New York (2019)
33. Templ, M., Gussenbauer, J., Filzmoser, P.: Evaluation of robust outlier detection methods for zero-inflated complex data. J. Appl. Stat. **47**(7), 1144–1167 (2020). https://doi.org/10.1080/02664763.2019.1671961
34. Tew, C., Giraud-Carrier, C., Tanner, K., Burton, S.: Behavior-based clustering and analysis of interestingness measures for association rule mining. Data Min. Knowl. Disc. **28**, 1004–1045 (2014)
35. Tukey, J.W.: Exploratory Data Analysis. Addison-Wesley, Boston (1977)
36. Webber, W., Moffat, A., Zobel, J.: A similarity measure for indefinite rankings. ACM Trans. Inf. Syst. **28**(4) (2010). https://doi.org/10.1145/1852102.1852106
37. Weiss, S.M., Kulikowski, C.A., Galen, R.S., Olsen, P.A., Natarajan, R.: Managing healthcare costs by peer-group modeling. Appl. Intell. **43**(4), 752–759 (2015). https://doi.org/10.1007/s10489-015-0685-7
38. Yang, J., Xie, M., Goh, T.: Outlier identification and robust parameter estimation in a zero-inflated poisson model. J. Appl. Stat. **38**, 421–430 (2011). https://doi.org/10.1080/02664760903456426

Improving Patient Trajectory Forecasts in Hospitals: Using Emergency Department Data for Length of Stay Prediction and Next Hospital Unit Classification

Alexander Winter[1,3], Toralf Kirsten[1], and Mattis Hartwig[2,3]

[1] Department of Medical Data Science, Leipzig University, Leipzig, Germany
alexander.winter@singular-it.de,
toralf.kirsten@medizin.uni-leipzig.de
[2] German Research Center for Artificial Intelligence, 23562 Lübeck, Germany
[3] singularIT GmbH, 04109 Leipzig, Germany
mattis.hartwig@dfki.de

Abstract. Accurately forecasting a patient's trajectory during hospitalization is essential for effective hospital management. Predicting length of stay (LOS) and next hospital unit can assist in resource planning and management, benefiting patients, physicians, and hospitals. This paper extends previous research on LOS prediction and introduces the task of next hospital unit classification. The study utilizes the MIMIC dataset, which now includes specific emergency department (ED) data, making it suitable for machine learning methodologies. Several contributions are made, including the addition of the next hospital unit classification task, an extended related work section, an expanded dataset description, and a thorough error analysis. The CatBoost model is employed to handle the high-dimensional categorical features in the dataset, along with feature engineering, hyperparameter tuning, and a customized loss function for the LOS regression task. Benchmarking against baseline models and related research demonstrates the superior performance of the proposed methods, with an average absolute error of 2.36 days for LOS prediction and a 50% accuracy for the next hospital unit classification. The paper provides a comprehensive overview of the related work, dataset description, approach, results, and concludes with insights and future directions.

Keywords: Length of stay prediction · Next hospital unit classification · Emergency department · Hospital management · Forecasting · MIMIC dataset · CatBoost model

1 Introduction

The capability to accurately predict a patient's trajectory during their hospitalization is crucial for effective hospital management. Forecasts of this nature can facilitate effective resource planning and management within the hospital, leading to benefits for patients, physicians, and the hospitals themselves [34]. Predicting a patient's length of stay (LOS) or a next hospital unit are two such cases in which a part of a patient's trajectory is forecast. Because of the high clinical value of such forecasts, various LOS prediction [17,30,34] and some next hospital unit cases have been researched [3,16]. Given that a large number of patients are admitted through the emergency department (ED), the transition phase from the ED to subsequent units represents a valuable opportunity for predicting the remaining LOS or the next hospital unit [10]. Fortunately, the rather recently published version 4 of the MIMIC dataset now includes specific ED data. Previous versions of the MIMIC dataset have been utilized in other LOS prediction research, allowing for comparability with our results [17,30]. With over 180,000 ED admissions, the MIMIC dataset presents a substantial data source well-suited for machine learning methodologies.

This paper is an extension of the conference paper "Predicting Hospital LOS of Patients Leaving the Emergency Department" published in the proceedings of the International Conference on Health Informatics 2023 [37]. We made several additional contributions which are detailed out in the following:

- **Additional Prediction Task.** We added the task of next hospital unit classification as an additional prediction task that can be run in parallel with the LOS regression.
- **Extended Related Work Section.** We restructured the related work section, added further literature on the LOS prediction task and added a paragraph on the next hospital unit prediction.
- **Extended Data Set Description.** We included additional descriptions of the subject demographics in our dataset, like average age and ethnicity.
- **Extended Error Analysis.** We examined relevant errors, which occurred during our experiments more thoroughly, to achieve a better understanding of the characteristics of cases with large prediction errors.
- **Overall Restructuring and Detailing.** We modified the structure of the paper to accommodate all the content changes mentioned above in this list. Additionally we added contextual details and extended the paper from 8 to 24 pages.

The MIMIC dataset is populated with numerous high-dimensional categorical features. To handle these, we utilize the state-of-the-art CatBoost model [14] for both prediction tasks, combined with a feature engineering and hyperparameter tuning. Furthermore, we've implemented a tailored loss function for the LOS regression task that has been successfully applied in other models [30]. For benchmarking we compared our predictions with both naive prediction models (e.g. mean or most common unit predictors) and comparable research from different but related use cases. Our methods resulted in an average absolute error of 2.36 days, which showcases a notable improvement over the baseline models, and holds up well when compared to the results of other prediction tasks using the MIMIC dataset. The classification task achieved a 50% accuracy and improved on each metric compared to the baseline models.

The remainder of the paper is structured as follows: Sect. 2 gives an overview of the related work when it comes to LOS prediction. The data set is introduced in Sect. 3 by giving an overview of the available data, some statistics and basic plots. Section 4 describes the approach for LOS prediction while Sect. 5 covers the next hospital unit classification. The results are discussed in Sect. 6. The paper concludes in Sect. 7.

2 Related Work

There are diverse applications of machine learning techniques in the hospital domain. Examples are improved diagnostics, better treatments and process optimization. In the process optimization area, LOS of patients has received special attention and thus has been researched from various perspectives. Sadler et al. [31] have identified LOS as a relevant business factor for the commercial performance of hospitals, De Jong et al. [11] have looked into the effect of LOS distributions in hospitals on doctor's decision making and Buttgieg et al. [5] have investigated structural effects that increase the overall average LOS for hospitals.

The research on predicting LOS started around 1959 with analyzing influencing factors of LOS for psychiatric patients [4,27]. Within ten years of research the first statistical models where build [18,29]. Since then LOS predictions have been performed with different models and datasets. For an extensive overview of studies connected to LOS prediction, Stone et al. [34] and Bacchi et al. [2] have set-up two review papers. Both review papers differentiate between solving a classification task (i. e. long vs short stay) and a regression task (i. e. predicting the LOS on a continuous time-scale). Many studies focus on specific datasets or cohorts of patients with common features. Launay et al. [24] have classified prolonged LOS using a neural network and Chang et al. [8] have further focused on classifying the prolonged LOS on severe subgroups in the data and have achieved best results using a CatBoost model. Zolbanin et al. [40] have focused on predicting LOS for patients with chronic diseases on a specialized dataset. Stone et al. [35] have focused on using admission data to predict the ED LOS. Several authors focus on using information from a previous unit to predict LOS of the next unit. Despite the importance of the patients that have come through ED admission, to our knowledge predicting LOS of patients from information available at the point in time of leaving the ED unit has not been researched before.

In this paper, we use the MIMIC-IV dataset [22], a collection of electronic health records (see next section for more information regarding the dataset itself). The MIMIC dataset (including older versions) has been used for all different kinds of health informatics tasks. Examples are predicting in-hospital mortality [20,25,26], predicting sepsis and septic shocks [13,33] or assessing a risk of treatments [12,21]. For further tasks see the review paper by Syed et al. [36].

The MIMIC dataset also has been used for LOS prediction. There are several papers that also have performed LOS prediction in other scenarios on older versions of the MIMIC dataset. Gentimis et al. [17] have set-up a binary classifier that differentiates between short ($\leq$ 5 days) and long ($>$ 5 days) stays after a patient leaves the intensive care unit (ICU) using a neural network. Zebin et al. [39] have used a similar approach with slightly different classes ($\leq$ 7 days and $>$ 7 days). Rocheteau et al. [30] have used a temporal pointwise convolutional model to predict the remaining days of patients in intensive care.

None of these papers have researched the task of predicting hospital LOS after an emergency department admission. An explanation is that the ED module was newly introduced in the MIMIC-IV version which was published rather recently. Even tough they have other focuses we use the papers by Gentimis et al. [17], Zebin et al. [39] and

Rocheteau et al. [30] as our core benchmarks for following sections to measure how our prediction performs compared to the performance of related tasks.

The second application that is covered in this paper is predicting the next unit after an emergency department admission. As described above predicting the next station can help hospitals plan the resources and capacities better. In general, that is a classification task which has similarities to other patient classification tasks e.g. predicting a treatment [19] or predicting a mortality [20]. To the best of our understanding, there has been no direct prediction made regarding the subsequent unit following an emergency department visit. However, Fernandes et al. [16] conducted a classification study on whether patients are transferred to the intensive care unit after being admitted to the emergency department.

As a final note, of course the conference paper that was the prework of this journal paper is also related work [37].

3 Dataset

This section provides information about the dataset used during the experiments. We introduce MIMIC-IV and further examine our cohort. We will also present an overview of the cohort features and discuss the methods used during the feature extraction and feature engineering.

3.1 MIMIC-IV

Our study is based on MIMIC-IV, a centralized medical information mart, which holds real-world health records of more than 250,000 patients having had a total of more than 520,000 admissions to the Beth Israel Deaconess Medical Center in Boston between the years 2008–2019 [22]. The database adopts a relational structure and has been designed to facilitate data analysis for researchers. Furthermore, all data has been deidentified according to the Health Insurance Portability and Accountability Act, protecting critical personal information of patients.

The MIMIC-IV database is structured into the modules *core*, *hosp* and *icu*, which store a comprehensive view of each patient stay from demographic information to laboratory results. The newly added *ed* module further includes data originating from the emergency department.

We have selected the cohort to only include stays of adult patients (age > 18), who entered the hospital through the emergency department. Additionally, we exclude very long stays (LOS > 50 days) to remove extreme outliers, which resulted in dropping 537 stays. Missing data is only present in the triage table in about eight percent of the total hospital stays. In order not to influence the final prediction by imputing data, we have decided to drop the stays from the final dataset. The selection resulted in a total of 181,797 individual hospital stays extracted from MIMIC-IV.

As Fig. 1 shows, ages are in the range of 18 to 91, with all patients older than 89 grouped into the age of 91. The largest amount of patients fall into the range of 50 to 70 years of age, with an average age of around 57 years of age. Women and men are distributed fairly equal in the dataset, with around 52% of stays by female patients.

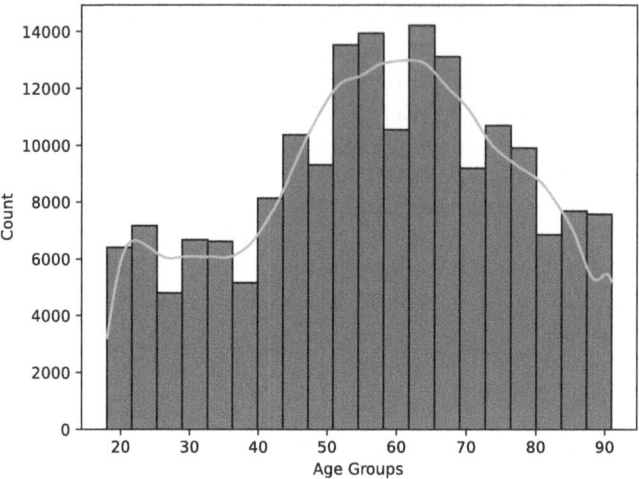

Fig. 1. Age distribution of the created dataset used for LOS prediction. Ages are grouped into ranges of 4 years. The kernel density estimation (yellow) provides complementary information about the shape of the age distribution [37] (Color figure online).

Patient ethnicity is reported in categories White, African American, Hispanic, Asian, American Indian, Unknown and Unable To Obtain, with the largest portion of 66% belonging to the category White.

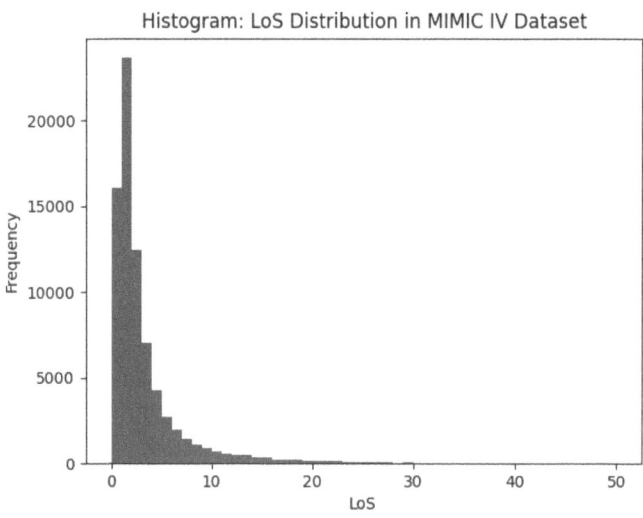

Fig. 2. LOS distribution as a histogram for all hospital stays from MIMIC-IV. Values larger than 50 are ignored for the purpose of visibility [37].

Figure 2 shows the LOS distribution for hospital stays in the MIMIC-IV database. The graph displays the typical positive skew of LOS data, with the mean at 3.9 days and a median value of 2.4 days.

MIMIC-IV uses categorical values in the *transfers* table to track the hospital units patients are transferred to. Here, each transfer a patient has during their stay is documented, including the unit where they came from and the unit which they are send to. In total, there are 41 different units to which a patient can be send to after the emergency department. Figure 3 shows an example transfer graph for patients with pneumonia (ICD code J18), which displays the units and frequencies of hospital transfers.

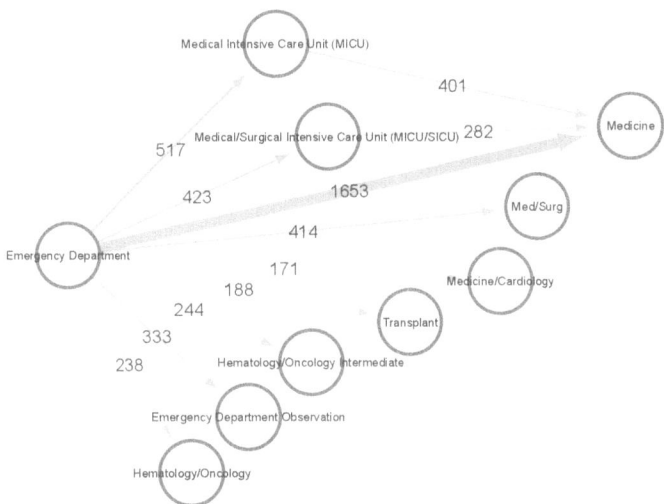

Fig. 3. Transfer graph for the specific ICD code J18 (Pneumonia). Nodes are hospital units which are connected by edges representing patient transfers. The number attached to an edge represents the patient transfer frequency between the ED and the follow up hospital unit.

3.2 Features

We categorize our features into the thematic groups demographics, medical and triage based on the research of Buttgieg et al. [5].

Demographics: are directly related to patients and their living circumstances. The data consists of the *age*, *gender*, *insurance* and *ethnicity*. The values are retrieved directly from the *patients* and *admission* table, as they are included in the electronic health record (EHR).

Medical: features refer to attributes that depend on the specific hospital stay. This includes the admission location providing information about the patients location before being admitted to the hospital and the diagnosis given to patients at the end of their emergency department stay in form of an ICD code.

By transformation of existing data, we have engineered additional features to take advantage of additional information existing in MIMIC-IV. The variables *los* and *ed_los* are based on the admission and discharge times from the hospital and emergency department. Using the admission and discharge times found in the *admission* and the *ed_stays* table, a timespan for the stay can be calculated directly for both values. They represent the fractional days a patient has spent in the hospital and the emergency department respectively. The *los* variable acts as the target variable for the task of LOS prediction.

The feature *careunit* is the target value for the hospital unit classification and is calculated by querying the MIMIC-IV *transfers* table. The table contains detailed information about all units a patient has visited during their stay. Querying the *eventtype* column by the keyword "admit" and selecting the care unit results in the first unit a patient has been admitted to after leaving the ED. Figure 3 is a graphical representation of such transfers.

The *diagnosis* table holds each diagnosis a patient received during their ED stay. Counting each diagnosis per stay resulted in the variable *diagnosis_count*. The variable *medicine_count* follows the same procedure, but is calculated from the *medrecon* table, which tracks the medicine a patient is taking currently. Both values are created to add further information about the complexity of the patients condition.

By counting the number of different hospital admissions for a single patient prior to the current admission date, we calculated the variable *previous_stays*. The variable *previous_stays_average_length* is created by adding the LOS value of the stays found and dividing by the number of previous stays.

Triage data is related to the patient's current health status and is collected while they are in the emergency department by a care provider, who first asks a series of questions to asses the patients condition. Afterwards the patient's vital signs are measured. Based on the measurement, the level of acuity is decided, which serves as the basis when deciding if the patient has to be put into critical care. Features resulting from vital signs are *resprate*, the respiratory rate in breaths per minute, *temperature*, *o2sat*, *sbp* and *dbp*, *paint* and *acuity*.

Table 1 gives an overview about all the features extracted from MIMIC-IV, including each type and where it is extracted from.

4 Length of Stay Prediction

In this section, we give a brief overview of the technical methodology used for the LOS prediction. The methodology is structured into the CatBoost architecture, the chosen loss functions and the hyperparameter tuning.

4.1 CatBoost Architecture

CatBoost is a gradient boosting, open-source library. It was developed to address the challenges that occur when handling categorical data. While conventional approaches require categorical data to be converted into a numerical representation manually, Cat-Boost is designed to handle categorical data directly [14]. Categorical data is handled by

Table 1. Features extracted from MIMIC-IV, with type and source table [37].

Group	Feature	Type	Source Table
Demographic	Gender	Binary	Patients
	Age	Discrete	Patients
	Ethnicity	Categorical	Admissions
	Insurance	Categorical	Admissions
Medical	ICD Code	Categorical	Diagnosis
	Adm. Location	Categorical	Admissions
	Diagnosis Count	Discrete	Engineered
	Medicine Count	Discrete	Engineered
	Previous Stays	Discrete	Engineered
	Prev. Stays Avg	Continuous	Engineered
	ED LoS	Continuous	Engineered
	LoS	Continous	Engineered
	Careunit	Categorical	Engineered
Triage	Resprate	Discrete	Triage
	Temperature	Continuous	Triage
	O2sat	Discrete	Triage
	sbp	Discrete	Triage
	dbp	Discrete	Triage
	Pain	Discrete	Triage
	Acuity	Discrete	Triage

calculating target statistics for each categorical feature, transforming them into numerical values and keeping the underlying information intact. CatBoost therefore avoids adding an extensive amount of columns to a dataset, a known drawback with One-Hot-Encoding [7]. The library becomes particularly useful in scenarios involving categorical features with a high cardinality. With over 13,000 different ICD codes in the database, the MIMIC-IV dataset presents an ideal opportunity to take advantage of the efficiency of CatBoost.

Compared to other, popular boosting frameworks like XGBoost [9] or LightGBM [23], CatBoost achieves state-of-the-art performance, both on quality and speed. It outperformed both frameworks on multiple tasks [14]. In the realm of boosting frameworks, CatBoost has increased in popularity compared to the other libraries. Examples for the application of CatBoost in the healthcare sector are the use in predicting ICU mortality [32] and in forecasting if a patient will need mechanical ventilation during the hospital stay [38].

4.2 Loss Function and Evaluation Metrics

Because LOS data inherently has a high positive skew, it is important to take the skewness into account and to mitigate against it [30]. We have chosen to use the CatBoost model in two configurations. One is fitted on the root mean squared error (RMSE) loss function provided by the CatBoost library, a commonly used metric in regression, which penalizes larger error more heavily than smaller ones. The other one is fitted with the root mean squared logarithmic error (RMSLE), which penalizes proportional errors and is less affected by outliers. Rocheteau et al. [30] have already proven in their prediction scenario that the RMSLE was able to handle the skew better. Since CatBoost does not provide RMSLE as an optimization objective, we have implemented it ourselves using the custom objective interface.

The LOS prediction has been conducted in a similar manner to the works of Rocheteau et al. [30] and Gentimits et al. [17]. To achieve comparability in the results, we adopted the metrics used in the aforementioned works, namely the mean squared error (MSE), mean absolute percentage error (MAPE), mean absolute error (MAE), mean squared logarithmic error (MSLE) and the coefficient of determination ($R2$). For the case of using predictions to optimize clinical processes and capacity, the MAE and MAPE errors are the most important. Additionally, we converted the results of the regressor and the target variable into a categorical representation of short ($\hat{y} <= 5$) vs. long stays ($\hat{y} > 5$), making it comparable to the prediction performed by Gentimis et al. [17].

4.3 Hyperparameter Tuning

Since CatBoost is a library for gradient boosted trees, hyperparameters fall into the domain of tree-specific parameters. CatBoost provides an order of importance in the documentation[1], going from conventionally most influential parameters to the more case specific ones. First, we used the CatBoost regression model with default values, to check for initial overfitting and to get reasonable default values for each parameter.

Subsequently, we conducted a grid search by considering the most influential parameters: the learning rate, tree depth, and L2 regularization. The values for the grid search are determined based on the default values and recommendations provided in the CatBoost documentation. The evaluation metric guided the selection of parameters from the run yielding the optimal performance. Table 2 presents the selected hyperparameters.

Performing the grid search has shown, that adjusting the tree depth contributed the most to the emergence of under- or overfitting. Larger trees performed better on the training dataset, however lost performance when making predictions on the validation data. A sign that the model lost the ability to generalize on new data.

---

[1] https://catboost.ai/en/docs/concepts/parameter-tuning.

Table 2. Hyperparameter selection of the final CatBoost model, after the grid search has been performed [37].

Hyperparameter	Value	Default
Learning rate	0.1	no
Tree Depth	6	no
L2 regularization	50	no
Random strength	1	yes
Bagging temperature	1	yes
Border count	128	yes
Internal dataset order	False	yes
Tree growing policy	Symmetric	yes

4.4 Generation of Final Results

The LOS prediction is performed with the model setup described above. We split our dataset into train, validation and test data with a proportion of 60%, 20% and 20% respectively. The training and testing is conducted in 10 runs, where each run has the model train and predict on a new, randomly sampled dataset, which introduces some randomness in the data to not influence the model training by a biased selection of the dataset.

To provide an unbiased evaluation of the model performance during training and hyperparameter tuning, the validation data is used to calculate the metrics during training. Finally, the model is tested on the new, unseen test data, where the evaluation metrics described in Sect. 4.2 are calculated from the model results.

To understand the impact of the diagnosis a patient received at the end of the emergency department stay, we have created two separate training datasets with varying levels of detail of the ICD code.

3 Digit ICD Code. The first dataset has the ICD codes truncated to 3 digit codes to reduce the cardinality, while also reducing the amount of information the ICD code holds.

Full ICD Code. The second dataset uses full ICD codes, where each ICD codes encodes the most information about the patients condition.

The separation has been performed to take advantage of CatBoosts ability to handle inputs with high cardinality. We calculate the selected evaluation metrics (see Sect. 4.2) based on the results of each run and calculate 95%-confidence for every metric. The same procedure is repeated for the baseline models.

4.5 Baselines

We included additional baseline models in our work, to evaluate the CatBoost model. We used mean and median predictors, which calculate the mean and median of the training dataset and use those values for every prediction. In our case the values are 3.9

for the mean and 2.4 for the median regressor. The so called dummy regressor is the most simple model possible, which is better than random guessing, because it is independent from the actual input when making a prediction. It is used to set performance expectations for the task on our specific dataset.

Additionally, we used a linear regression model to predict the LOS as a further baseline. Linear regression has been used in LOS prediction before and is usually a popular choice, because it is widely applicable and the results can be easily interpreted [1].

5 Hospital Unit Classification

We further examine the usability of ED data as a planning tool for hospitals by predicting the hospital unit a patient is sent to after they leave the emergency department. The classifier architecture, training process and methodology of the experiments are described in this section.

5.1 Model and Evaluation Metrics

The classification model is designed in a very similar way to the regressor described in Sect. 4. The goal of the classifier is to predict the unit a patient will be sent to after their stay in the ED, only using data collected from the particular stay. CatBoost provides algorithms for both classification and regression tasks. The architecture therefore does not need to be altered in any way. A simple change of the model from the CatBoost regressor to the CatBoost classifier was sufficient. We use the CatBoost classifier with the multi-class prediction setup, as we want the model to be able to select between various different hospital units. The dataset has 41 different units, a patient can be admitted to after leaving the ED. The final prediction is a list of probabilities for each unit in the testing dataset. From the list, the accuracy for the most likely unit can be inferred, as well as other metrics like the top-N accuracy.

The metrics in use for the classification task are the accuracy, precision and recall. They are selected, because they give a good initial understanding of how well the model is performing overall in making predictions. Comparing these values to the defined baseline models makes it possible to evaluate the models performance. Furthermore, the-top-three and top-five-accuracy are used as a performance metric. In multi-class classification accuracy can drop significantly, because it is an additional challenge for the model to get every class label perfectly right. Looking at top-N -accuracy can help to put the results of the stricter metrics into perspective.

5.2 Hyperparameter Selection

The process of hyperparameter tuning is analogous to the selection of hyperparameters for the regressor. For multi-class classification CatBoost does not set the learning rate automatically. It is set to 0.1 for the initial run. Again after about 1,000 iterations, the model did not improve any further, therefore this value is used for the grid search. Here we chose the same values as mentioned in Sect. 4.3.

Although the model also did not improve past a certain threshold, the alteration of the parameters did have a more pronounced effect on the outputs of the model. The emergence of overfitting can be observed when raising the tree sizes and the learning rate. Larger trees show a great divergence between the test and training loss, which means even though they are able to capture more information about the training data, they are not able to generalize onto unseen samples.

5.3 Generation of Final Results

The training pipeline is setup analogously to the LOS prediction experiment. We used the same proportion for our dataset splits and performed the training and testing again in 10 distinct runs. The same dataset can be utilized for both models, with minor differences. The target variable has been transformed into a multi-class prediction, where the admission location serves as the target class. The LOS value has been removed completely, since it is unknown at the point of leaving the ED. No further alterations have been made to the datasets. The workflow is analogous to the regressor model, with the only difference being the prediction, which the model outputs at the end. The output is a list of probabilities of the classes the model has encountered during training, ranging from the most likely class at first place to the most unlikely last. Again, two datasets are used for training the classifier and predicting the next hospital unit.

Grouped Care Unit. There are 41 different stations in the MIMIC-IV dataset, while many occur only less than two percent in the total transfers. In order to balance the label distribution, the stations are grouped into the ten stations with the highest occurence and the label *other*, which summarizes the stations with very few samples in the dataset.

All Care Units. All stations are included as retrieved from MIMIC-IV. This dataset is used to evaluate the impact of the aggregation on the different models.

5.4 Baselines

Similar to regression, a straightforward baseline approach for classification involves disregarding the input entirely and consistently returning a fixed value. This approach is implemented through a dummy classifier. We use two distinct configurations of the dummy classifier. The first configuration considers the labels present in the training data and always predicts the class that occurs most frequently. The second configuration is based on random guessing, where each observed label during training is assigned an equal probability of being selected as the predicted label.

Another simple, yet popular approach is the K-nearest neighbors classification. Here, data is classified based on the distances of data points inside the feature space. It is assumed that data points close to each other are similar and therefore belong to the same class. When classifying a new test input x, first the Euclidean Distances[2] to the K neighboring points are calculated. The labels of the selected data points are counted and the new point gets assigned to the class which occurred the most often. K-nearest neighbors classification is a simple, but effective approach, which can be easily set up

---
[2] Other distance measures can be used as well. We focus on the one most commonly used.

and does not require any hyperparameter tuning. The only parameter, that has to be set is K itself. A common approach for the selection of a number K is to plot the errors of different values and select the one which minimizes the error. By performing a grid search over predefined values for K, we selected $K = 3$ as the optimal value, since there was no further improvement in accuracy.

6 Results and Discussion

In this section, we present the results of the models performing LOS prediction and compare our results and accuracy metrics to related works [17, 30]. Furthermore, we showcase the outcomes of the hospital unit classification and compare the metrics of the classification model to the selected baselines.

6.1 Length of Stay Prediction

The selected metrics for seven different regressor models are shown in Table 3. The three initial models serve as baseline models. The median model, which constantly predicts lower LOS times, has a slightly worse performance on the MSE due to the skewed nature of the LOS curve. However, when looking at the primary metrics in terms of usability, MAE and MAPE are better choices of metrics for the median model. The linear regression on the other hand, did not contribute any value, in fact worsens the models performance. This highlights the necessity for a more complex model to solve the given use case.

The four models presented in the bottom part of the table are different configurations of the CatBoost model, each having been trained on two distinct datasets. Notably, all four models outperform the baseline models. Among the models, the CatBoost (RMSLE, 3-digit ICD codes) achieves the best results for the MAE with 2.36 and a

Table 3. Regression results of the CatBoost model compared to the defined baselines. Three separate datasets are used during the experiments and the metrics are calculated for each dataset. The CatBoost model is trained with both the RMSE and RMSLE loss function. For the first four metrics lower values indicate a better prediction performance. The R2 score is optimal for a value of one. We calculated the 95% confidence intervals for each metric from 10 runs. The variation was very small, we therefore chose to omit it in the table [37].

Model	MSE	MAE	MAPE	MSLE	R2
Mean	25.03	3.15	372	0.66	0
Median	27.60	2.88	229	0.57	−0.09
Linear Regression	27.30	3.34	379	0.73	−0.09
CatBoost (RMSE) (3 digit ICD code)	20.23	2.61	209	0.42	0.18
CatBoost (RMSLE) (3 digit ICD code)	21.59	2.36	136	0.36	0.13
CatBoost (RMSE) (Full ICD code)	19.82	2.58	206	0.41	0.18
CatBoost (RMSLE) (Full ICD code)	21.70	2.42	129	0.36	0.11

MAPE of 136. While the results represent a significant increase compared to the baselines, there is still room for improvement. The adoption of the RMSLE loss function proved to be advantageous, as it achieved a significant gain compared to the RMSE loss function. The boost in performance aligns with other research in use cases with skewed distributions in the prediction variable [15,28,30]. Figure 4 visualizes the centralization of the prediction error around zero, with around 43 percent of errors being below one day. As negative values signify underpredictions, the overall shift to the right implies a tendency of the model trained with the RMSLE loss function to overpredict. The model predictions are very stable over the ten runs and the confidence intervals have therefore been omitted from Table 3.

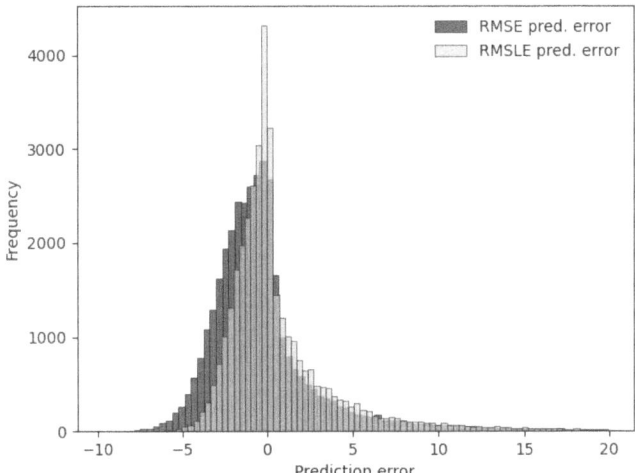

Fig. 4. Comparison of prediction errors for the RMSE (blue) and RMSLE (light-blue) loss functions. RMSLE has a lower variance, further centering the errors around zero. Predictions errors that are greater than 20 days are hidden here, to improve readability [37] (Color figure online).

The feature importance obtained from the CatBoost library is shown in Fig. 5. The figure shows that the top features are all related directly to the patient condition, with the most important feature being the actual diagnosis. Additionally, the significant impact of engineered features can be highlighted, as four out of the top ten features have been created by feature engineering techniques. Worth noting however is the high influence of the ed_los variable, which can be influenced by a multitude of factors unrelated to the patient condition. For example holding patients in the ED because of hospital unit overcrowding, would prolong the ED stay as well. Consequently, the exact composition of the ed_los and its actual influence on the hospital LOS should be further investigated.

Finally, the graph shows that the model assigns a higher importance to the medical features, which are related to the patient condition directly. Among the features, the ICD code had the overall largest impact and significantly influenced the final prediction. Comparing the results on the two datasets from Table 3 shows an increase in

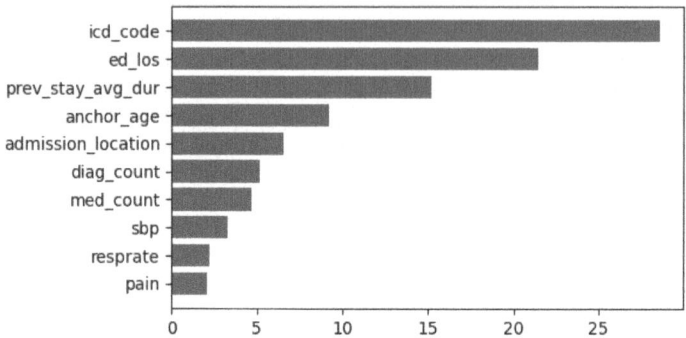

Fig. 5. Top 10 most important features to the CatBoost model. Each bar shows how much on average the prediction changes if the feature value is altered. The importance is normalized to equal 100 [37].

performance when using the full ICD code, which further confirms the importance of accounting for categorical data.

Table 4. Performance of the regressor model compared to the works of Rocheateau et al. [30], Zebin et al. [39] and Gentimis et al. [17]. The same metrics are used for comparison [37].

Model	MSE	MAE	MAPE	MSLE	R2	Short vs. Long
CatBoost (RMSE)	20.23	2.61	209.0	0.42	0.18	74%
CatBoost (RMSLE)	21.59	2.36	136.0	0.36	0.13	78%
TPC (MSE)	21.60	2.21	154.3	1.80	0.27	—
TPC (MSLE)	21.70	1.78	63.5	0.70	0.27	—
Gentimis NN	—	—	—	—	—	79%
Zebin Autoencoder+DNN	—	—	—	—	—	78%

As mentioned above, the results from Rocheteau et al. [30], Gentimis et al. [17] and Zebin et al. [39] serve as comparison works for our results. Although the works use data different to our ED use case and solved different prediction tasks, we wanted to include a comparison to verify, if our performance metrics are in a similar range. Gentimis et al. [17] predict the LOS of the patients after they leave the ICU. Rocheteau et al. [30] predict the time the patients are staying in ICU. And finally Zebin et al. [39] classify for short or long ICU stays by using data obtained within 24 h of admission.

To measure the performance of the model, we have chosen the same metrics as selected by Rocheteau et al. [30]. However, Gentimis et al. [17] and Zebin et al. [39] approached the prediction task differently by classifying stays as long or short. In order to facilitate a fair comparison, we transformed the prediction outputs of the CatBoost model retroactively, depending on its value being above or below 5 days. We calculated accuracy by comparing these transformed values to the results of the benchmarking papers.

Table 4 displays the results of all metrics, including the accuracy of classifying short stays versus long stays. Albeit slightly inferior compared to the Temporal Pointwise Convolution Network created by Rocheteau et al. in terms of MAE and MAPE, the CatBoost model yielded similar results in the MSE. The distribution of ICU LOS is significantly narrower compared to regular station LOS after ED dismissal which might be part of the explanation. Additionally, the observation made by Rocheteau et al. regarding the improvement in performance when transitioning from RMSE/MSE to RMSLE/MSLE can also be seen in our results. Our transformed classification metric shows almost identical accuracy performance (78% for the CatBoost RMSLE, 3-Digit Groups) as the results of Gentimis et al. (79%) and Zebin et al. (77.7%).

6.2 Next Hospital Unit Classification

The results of the second experiment are displayed in Table 5. The model is tested on two different datasets, one where the target label contains all available care units in MIMIC-IV with a total of 36 and one where rare units are grouped into the category *Other*, which resulted in 11 total categories. Again, the CatBoost model outperformed every baseline model for every metric on both datasets. The dummy regressor has the worst overall performance, with accuracy, precision, recall and F1-Score being the same for both datasets, since the most frequent class is unchanged. The Top-3 and Top-5-Accuracy are significantly worse for the fully labeled dataset. The K-nearest neighbors method improved upon the dummy regressor for each metric, except for accuracy and recall, which dropped slightly. Comparing the baselines to the CatBoost model shows a large improvement of around 50% of the second best score for the first four metrics. The multi-class specific metrics also increased for the CatBoost classifier, with around 75% of labels being in the top three predictions. Comparing the two datasets reveals that grouping the labels only leads to a slight gain in prediction performance. Every metric only increased by around five to eight percent for the grouped dataset.

Figure 6 shows the predicted labels as frequencies. The most commonly predicted care units are Emergency Department Observation, Medicine and Other, which make up a total of 90% of the total predictions. Table 6 illustrates a confusion matrix of the model predictions, which shows a clear imbalance in the frequency among hospital units. One can see that the model rarely predicted classes that did not have a high support in the training dataset. The cells along the diagonal represent the correctly classified instances,

Table 5. Results of the CatBoost classifier against the respective baselines. Each model has been trained and tested on two datasets.

Data	Model	Accuracy	Precision	Recall	F1 Score	Top 3 Acc	Top 5 Accuracy
Grouped Careunit	CatBoost	0.49	0.46	0.49	0.43	0.76	0.88
	Dummy Classifier	0.27	0.07	0.27	0.12	0.46	0.55
	K-nearest neighbors	0.26	0.22	0.26	0.22	0.50	0.60
All Careunits	CatBoost	0.45	0.41	0.45	0.38	0.68	0.80
	Dummy Classifier	0.27	0.07	0.27	0.12	0.3	0.34
	K-nearest neighbors	0.24	0.18	0.24	0.20	0.40	0.42

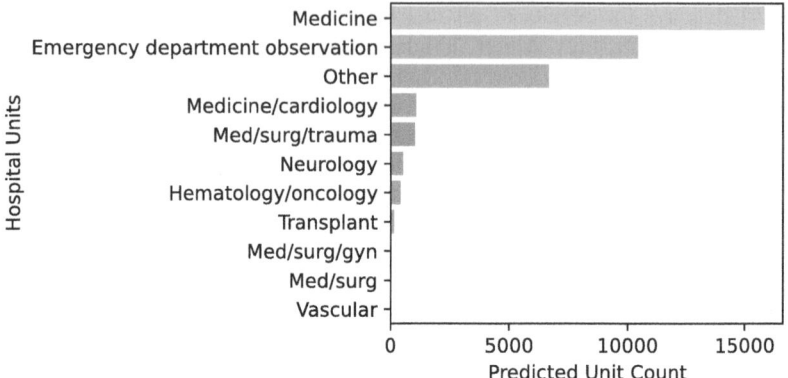

Fig. 6. Visualization of the classification results.

while off-diagonal cells represent misclassifications. The maximum values (blue) are mostly off-diagonal, indicating that the actual classes and predicted classes are not correlated strongly. The classification is incorrect for most classes, since the model mostly predicted the three classes Emergency Department Observation, Medicine and Other.

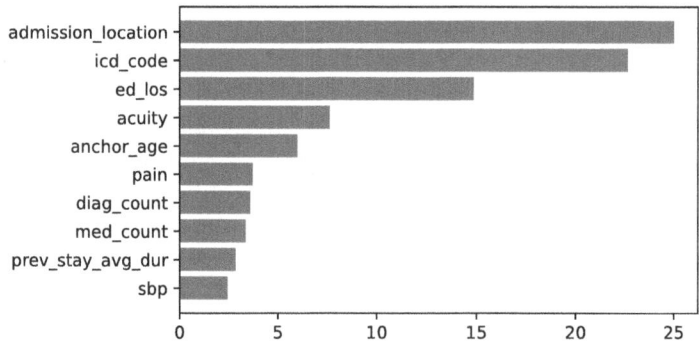

Fig. 7. Top 10 most important features to the CatBoost Classifier.

Inspecting the values of each column, one can see how the predictions of a particular class are distributed among the actual classes. Here, the maximum values of the column for each predicted class belong to the target unit, meaning that the predictions for certain classes were mostly correct. Therefore, even though there are many misclassifications, the model still captured the overall trend for predicting the actual classes.

A large part of the missing performance displayed in the evaluation metrics can be attributed to the imbalance in the dataset. Since the classifier can be seen as a recommender system, giving a suggestion to which unit a patient most likely will be send to, the meaningfulness of evaluating only the top class can be questioned.

Table 6. Confusion matrix of the Next Unit Classification. Rows represent the actual hospital unit, while columns represent the predicted class. The values have been normalized by rows, resulting in the proportion of instances predicted as a particular class compared to the true instances of this class. The values are given in percent.

	ED Obs	Hematology	Surg	GYN	Trauma	Medicine	Cardiology	Neurology	Transplant	Vascular	Other
ED Obs	83.11	0.10	0.00	0.06	0.89	11.42	0.99	0.27	0.04	0.00	3.10
Hematology	8.37	12.90	0.31	0.08	1.77	66.21	0.92	0.77	0.46	0.00	8.22
Surg	11.99	1.36	0.54	0.25	5.43	66.35	1.77	1.48	0.47	0.03	10.32
GYN	13.70	2.59	0.08	1.70	4.78	66.77	0.65	1.05	0.16	0.00	8.51
Trauma	15.66	0.94	0.65	0.29	27.85	46.56	0.36	0.22	0.07	0.00	7.40
Medicine	8.42	0.83	0.04	0.07	1.74	71.06	1.51	0.72	0.32	0.05	15.26
Cardiology	11.66	0.27	0.00	0.00	0.00	29.85	27.32	2.33	0.20	0.13	28.25
Neurology	8.80	0.71	0.00	0.06	2.07	42.92	3.42	12.81	0.35	0.06	28.81
Transplant	7.26	2.54	0.29	0.15	2.03	62.96	1.38	1.38	5.01	0.07	16.92
Vascular	8.17	1.08	0.09	0.00	3.50	55.75	11.49	3.23	0.27	0.36	16.07
Other	7.25	0.53	0.02	0.08	1.29	32.16	2.99	1.27	0.48	0.02	53.93

Observing the top-3- and top-5-accuracy provides a more balanced view of the performance of the CatBoost model. A significant increase to over 75% is visible for the top-3-accuracy and about 87% for the correct class being among the top-5 predicted labels. The visible increase shows that the model is able to learn the relationship between hospital units and the patient condition, increasing the prediction performance further compared to the baseline models.

The feature importance for the CatBoost Classifier presented in Fig. 7 shows a different trend to Fig. 5. While the *icd_code* and *ed_los* are important features for both models, the *admission_location* and *acuity* have a larger impact on the classification of the next unit.

6.3 Case Study: Evaluating Relevant Errors

To better understand the predictions and shortcomings of the models used during the experiments, we inspect the relevant errors in more detail. As presented in Fig. 8 the predictions centralize around the regression line for lower LOS values. While the model is able to adjust the predictions for longer stays, it is unable to predict the more extreme LOS values above 20 days correctly. Due to the high skew of LOS data, there are fewer cases available with extreme values, making it harder for the model to generalize on such cases, which is a common problem when predicting on EHRs [39].

In their assessment checklist for medical AI studies, Cabitza and Campagner [6] suggest to further explore the characteristics of relevant errors, for which the prediction error is much higher than the calculated metrics. As suggested, we inspect cases where the regression prediction is at least double the MAE. Around 10% of the predictions fall into this category.

Table 7 shows the difference between the relevant errors and errors, which are smaller than one day. Relevant errors show a remarkably high LOS average compared to the cases where the prediction error is small. Generally, the relevant errors are linked to cases with more severe patient conditions, which is confirmed by observing Fig. 9.

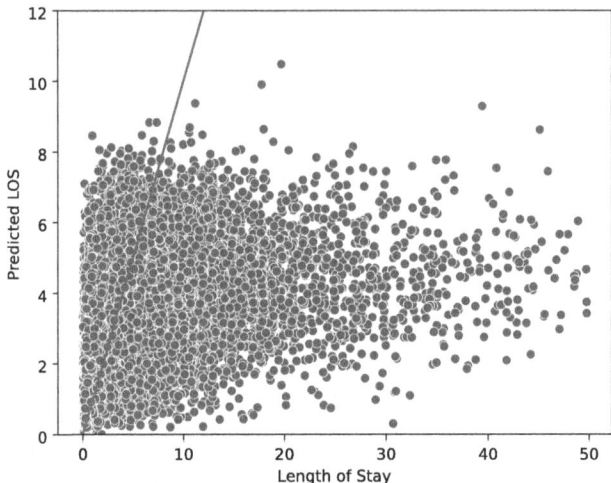

Fig. 8. Actual LOS compared to the predicted values. The regression line (red) represents data points where the prediction error would be zero. (Color figure online)

Table 7. Comparing relevant errors, where the prediction performance is poor, to the cases on which the predicted values are close to the target. Each column shows the average over all the cases belonging to the group.

	LOS	Age	Previous Stay Duration	Previous Stays
Relevant Errors (MAE $\geq$ 5)	14.9	60.1	2.9	2.3
Small Errors (MAE $\leq$ 1)	2.0	52.6	1.3	2.0

Here we compare three ICD codes on which the prediction performance was poor. The Codes translate into Heart Failure (I50.9), Sepsis (A41.9) and Disorder of brain (G93.9). The average absolute error for the aforementioned codes is at around four days and also contains a large variance. All of the diagnoses can generally be categorized as severe conditions, requiring intense medical attention. Based on the feature importance analysis presented in Fig. 5, it is evident that the predictions depend mostly on the given ICD code. With only 1.6% out of all the stays in the dataset being diagnosed with one of the above conditions, the total number of cases with severe conditions appears to be insufficient for the model to be able to generalize on such cases. Compared to a fairly common, less critical diagnosis like Anxiety disorder (F41.9), the predictions are much closer to the target, with an average error of less than 0.2 days.

Lastly, we inspect the relationship between the classification results and the predicted LOS. We let both models predict on the same testing dataset, merged the results for each case and grouped by the classification being correct or incorrect. Looking at the MAE for each group shows, that the wrongly classified cases also have a higher average regression error. For the correctly classified cases the MAE is around 1.92 and for the wrongly classified group it is 2.78.

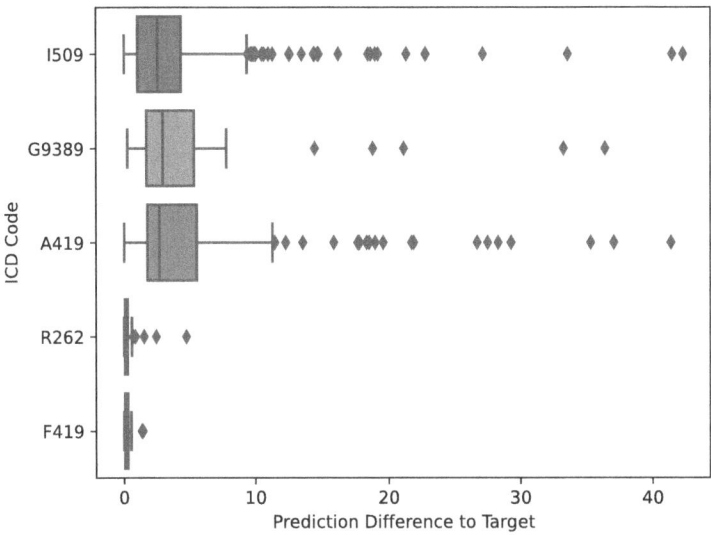

Fig. 9. Visualization of ICD codes on which the prediction performance is poor (Top 3) compared against ICD codes for which the performance is good (Bottom 2).

7 Conclusion

We evaluated the usability of ED data for process optimization in hospitals, by conducting two experiments on data selected from the MIMIC-IV dataset. The first entailed predicting the LOS of patients subsequent to their visit to the ED, while the second involved classifying the subsequent hospital unit a patient would be transferred to after the ED. These tasks were designed to rely solely on data accessible during a patient's ED visit.

We trained CatBoost models both for the LOS prediction and the next unit classification task, using the provided regressor and classifier setup respectively. For the regressor, we additionally implemented the MSLE loss function as a transfer from other models to the CatBoost architecture. Our prediction performance was better than the implemented baseline models for both tasks and comparable to similar use cases of predictions using the MIMIC dataset for LOS prediction. The performed feature engineering had a positive effect on the prediction quality, as 4 out of the top 10 important features are engineered, which further reiterates the importance of taking advantage of domain knowledge to extract additional information. The average absolute error of 2.36 days is a significant improvement compared to the baselines, as is the accuracy of around 50% during the classification of the next hospital unit. Additionally, our results are comparable with different but related use cases of LOS predictions.

Both experiments leave room for improvement. Analyzing relevant errors has revealed, that the regression performance is lower when predicting cases with a high LOS, usually linked to critical patient conditions. Connecting the predicted LOS to the classification results, shows that the MAE is worse, when the classification was incorrect. Due to the high skew of real-world LOS, the number of very long stays and accordingly the occurrence of critical diagnosis only accounts for a small part of the data. As aim to predict the critical conditions in a hospital setting, a further reduction of the prediction error based on our presented approach will be a target for future research. Potential ideas could be to refine the feature engineering process with more domain knowledge, e.g. by further grouping of high dimensional categorical features, or to benchmark further model architectures, e.g. Generalized Linear Models (GLMs) that have proven to be effective in dealing with skewed data.

References

1. Austin, P.C., Rothwell, D.M., Tu, J.V.: A comparison of statistical modeling strategies for analyzing length of stay after CABG surgery. Health Serv. Outcomes Res. Method. **3**(2), 107–133 (2002). https://doi.org/10.1023/a:1024260023851
2. Bacchi, S., Tan, Y., Oakden-Rayner, L., Jannes, J., Kleinig, T., Koblar, S.: Machine learning in the prediction of medical inpatient length of stay. Intern. Med. J. **52**(2), 176–185 (2022)
3. Bertsimas, D., Pauphilet, J., Stevens, J., Tandon, M.: Predicting inpatient flow at a major hospital using interpretable analytics. Manuf. Serv. Oper. Manag. **24**(6), 2809–2824 (2022)
4. Brown, G.: Social factors influencing length of hospital stay of schizophrenic patients. BMJ **2**(5162), 1300 (1959)
5. Buttigieg, S.C., Abela, L., Pace, A.: Variables affecting hospital length of stay: a scoping review. J. Health Organ. Manag. **32**(3), 463–493 (2018). https://doi.org/10.1108/jhom-10-2017-0275
6. Cabitza, F., Campagner, A.: The need to separate the wheat from the chaff in medical informatics: introducing a comprehensive checklist for the (self)-assessment of medical AI studies. Int. J. Med. Inform. **153**, 104510 (2021). https://doi.org/10.1016/j.ijmedinf.2021.104510. https://www.sciencedirect.com/science/article/pii/S1386505621001362
7. Cerda, P., Varoquaux, G.: Encoding high-cardinality string categorical variables. IEEE Trans. Knowl. Data Eng. **34**(3), 1164–1176 (2022). https://doi.org/10.1109/tkde.2020.2992529
8. Chang, Y.H., et al.: Machine learning-based triage to identify low-severity patients with a short discharge length of stay in emergency department. BMC Emerg. Med. **22**(1), 1–10 (2022)
9. Chen, T., Guestrin, C.: Xgboost: a scalable tree boosting system. CoRR abs/1603.02754 (2016). http://arxiv.org/abs/1603.02754
10. Christ, M., Grossmann, F., Winter, D., Bingisser, R., Platz, E.: Modern triage in the emergency department. Deutsches Ärzteblatt Int. 892–898 (2010). https://doi.org/10.3238/arztebl.2010.0892
11. De Jong, J.D., Westert, G.P., Lagoe, R., Groenewegen, P.P.: Variation in hospital length of stay: do physicians adapt their length of stay decisions to what is usual in the hospital where they work? Health Serv. Res. **41**(2), 374–394 (2006)
12. Dervishi, A.: Fuzzy risk stratification and risk assessment model for clinical monitoring in the ICU. Comput. Biol. Med. **87**, 169–178 (2017)
13. Desautels, T., et al.: Prediction of sepsis in the intensive care unit with minimal electronic health record data: a machine learning approach. JMIR Med. Inform. **4**(3), e5909 (2016)
14. Dorogush, A.V., Ershov, V., Gulin, A.: Catboost: gradient boosting with categorical features support. arXiv abs/1810.11363 (2018)
15. Feng, C., et al.: Log-transformation and its implications for data analysis. Shanghai Arch. Psychiatry **26**, 105–9 (2014). https://doi.org/10.3969/j.issn.1002-0829.2014.02.009

16. Fernandes, M., et al.: Predicting intensive care unit admission among patients presenting to the emergency department using machine learning and natural language processing. PLoS ONE **15**(3), e0229331 (2020)
17. Gentimis, T., Alnaser, A.J., Durante, A., Cook, K., Steele, R.: Predicting hospital length of stay using neural networks on MIMIC III data. In: 2017 IEEE 15th International Conference on Dependable, Autonomic and Secure Computing, 15th International Conference on Pervasive Intelligence and Computing, 3rd International Conference on Big Data Intelligence and Computing and Cyber Science and Technology Congress (DASC/PiCom/DataCom/CyberSciTech) (2017). https://doi.org/10.1109/dasc-picom-datacom-cyberscitec.2017.191
18. Gustafson, D.H.: Length of stay: prediction and explanation. Health Serv. Res. **3**(1), 12 (1968)
19. Heit, M., Rosenquist, C., Culligan, P., Graham, C., Murphy, M., Shott, S.: Predicting treatment choice for patients with pelvic organ prolapse. Obstet. Gynecol. **101**(6), 1279–1284 (2003)
20. Hou, N., et al.: Predicting 30-days mortality for MIMIC-III patients with sepsis-3: a machine learning approach using XGboost. J. Transl. Med. **18**(1), 1–14 (2020)
21. Huddar, V., Desiraju, B.K., Rajan, V., Bhattacharya, S., Roy, S., Reddy, C.K.: Predicting complications in critical care using heterogeneous clinical data. IEEE Access **4**, 7988–8001 (2016)
22. Johnsen, A., Bulgarelli, L., Horng, S., Celi, L.A., Mark, R.: MIMIC-IV (version 1.0) (2021). https://physionet.org/content/mimiciv/1.0/. https://doi.org/10.13026/s6n6-xd98
23. Ke, G., et al.: Lightgbm: a highly efficient gradient boosting decision tree. In: Guyon, I., et al. (eds.) Advances in Neural Information Processing Systems, vol. 30. Curran Associates, Inc. (2017). https://proceedings.neurips.cc/paper_files/paper/2017/file/6449f44a102fde848669bdd9eb6b76fa-Paper.pdf
24. Launay, C., Rivière, H., Kabeshova, A., Beauchet, O.: Predicting prolonged length of hospital stay in older emergency department users: use of a novel analysis method, the artificial neural network. Eur. J. Intern. Med. **26**(7), 478–482 (2015)
25. Li, F., Xin, H., Zhang, J., Fu, M., Zhou, J., Lian, Z.: Prediction model of in-hospital mortality in intensive care unit patients with heart failure: machine learning-based, retrospective analysis of the mimic-iii database. BMJ Open **11**(7), e044779 (2021)
26. Nowroozilarki, Z., Pakbin, A., Royalty, J., Lee, D.K., Mortazavi, B.J.: Real-time mortality prediction using MIMIC-IV ICU data via boosted nonparametric hazards. In: 2021 IEEE EMBS International Conference on Biomedical and Health Informatics (BHI), pp. 1–4. IEEE (2021)
27. Parnell, R., Skottowe, I.: Length of stay in mental hospitals and some factors influencing it. BMJ **2**(5162), 1296 (1959)
28. Rengasamy, D., Rothwell, B., Figueredo, G.P.: Asymmetric loss functions for deep learning early predictions of remaining useful life in aerospace gas turbine engines. In: 2020 International Joint Conference on Neural Networks (IJCNN), pp. 1–7 (2020). https://doi.org/10.1109/ijcnn48605.2020.9207051
29. Robinson, G.H., Davis, L.E., Leifer, R.P.: Prediction of hospital length of stay. Health Serv. Res. **1**(3), 287 (1966)
30. Rocheteau, E., Liò, P., Hyland, S.: Temporal pointwise convolutional networks for length of stay prediction in the intensive care unit. In: Proceedings of the Conference on Health, Inference, and Learning (2021). https://doi.org/10.1145/3450439.3451860
31. Sadler, B.L., et al.: Fable hospital 2.0: the business case for building better health care facilities. Hastings Cent. Rep. **41**(1), 13–23 (2011)

32. Safaei, N., et al.: E-catboost: an efficient machine learning framework for predicting ICU mortality using the EICU collaborative research database. PLoS ONE **17**(5) (2022). https://doi.org/10.1371/journal.pone.0262895
33. Scherpf, M., Gräßer, F., Malberg, H., Zaunseder, S.: Predicting sepsis with a recurrent neural network using the MIMIC III database. Comput. Biol. Med. **113**, 103395 (2019)
34. Stone, K., Zwiggelaar, R., Jones, P., Mac Parthaláin, N.: A systematic review of the prediction of hospital length of stay: towards a unified framework. PLOS Digit. Health **1**(4), e0000017 (2022)
35. Stone, K., Zwiggelaar, R., Jones, P., Parthaláin, N.M.: Predicting hospital length of stay for accident and emergency admissions. In: Ju, Z., Yang, L., Yang, C., Gegov, A., Zhou, D. (eds.) UKCI 2019. AISC, vol. 1043, pp. 283–295. Springer, Cham (2020). https://doi.org/10.1007/978-3-030-29933-0_24
36. Syed, M., et al.: Application of machine learning in intensive care unit (ICU) settings using mimic dataset: systematic review. Informatics **8**(1) (2021). https://doi.org/10.3390/informatics8010016. https://www.mdpi.com/2227-9709/8/1/16
37. Winter, A., Hartwig, M., Kirsten., T.: Predicting hospital length of stay of patients leaving the emergency department. In: Proceedings of the 16th International Joint Conference on Biomedical Engineering Systems and Technologies (BIOSTEC 2023) - HEALTHINF, pp. 124–131. INSTICC, SciTePress (2023). https://doi.org/10.5220/0011671700003414
38. Yu, L., et al.: Machine learning methods to predict mechanical ventilation and mortality in patients with covid-19. PLoS ONE **16**(4) (2021). https://doi.org/10.1371/journal.pone.0249285
39. Zebin, T., Rezvy, S., Chaussalet, T.J.: A deep learning approach for length of stay prediction in clinical settings from medical records. In: 2019 IEEE Conference on Computational Intelligence in Bioinformatics and Computational Biology (CIBCB), pp. 1–5. IEEE (2019)
40. Zolbanin, H.M., Davazdahemami, B., Delen, D., Zadeh, A.H.: Data analytics for the sustainable use of resources in hospitals: predicting the length of stay for patients with chronic diseases. Inf. Manag. 103282 (2020)

Suroy-Suroy: An Immersive Virtual Reality Therapy Game for Persons Living with Dementia in the Philippines

Veeda Michelle M. Anlacan[1,2,3], Angelo Cedric F. Panganiban[1,4(✉)], Roland Dominic G. Jamora[1,2], Isabel Teresa O. Salido[1], Romuel Aloizeus Z. Apuya[1], Bryan Andrei C. Galecio[1], Michael L. Tee[1,5], Maria Eliza R. Aguila[1,6], Cherica A. Tee[1,7], and Jaime D. L. Caro[1,4]

[1] Augmented Experience Ehealth Laboratory, University of the Philippines Manila, Manila, Philippines
axel@up.edu.ph
[2] Department of Neurosciences, College of Medicine - Philippine General Hospital, University of the Philippines Manila, Manila, Philippines
[3] Center for Memory and Cognition, Philippine General Hospital, University of the Philippines Manila, Manila, Philippines
[4] Department of Computer Science, College of Engineering, University of the Philippines Diliman, Quezon City, Philippines
afpanganiban@up.edu.ph
[5] Department of Physiology, College of Medicine, University of the Philippines Manila, Manila, Philippines
[6] Department of Physical Therapy, College of Allied Medical Professions, University of the Philippines Manila, Manila, Philippines
[7] Department of Pediatrics, College of Medicine, University of the Philippines Manila, Manila, Philippines
https://axel.upm.edu.ph/

Abstract. To aid in the need for alternative and non-pharmacological interventions for managing behavioral and psychological symptoms of dementia (BPSD), previous studies explored the utilization of immersive technologies such as virtual reality (VR). As part of these ongoing efforts, the researchers iteratively developed a VR game application in collaboration with Philippine healthcare professionals and scientists representing different fields of interest. This paper built upon previous works by further refining novel concepts and VR features for potential clinical evaluation. Additionally, this paper also provided comprehensive discussions on these concepts and techniques tailored for individuals living with dementia in the Philippines. These discussions could serve as a robust foundation for future development and overall adoption of VR -based interventions in this context. With the versatility of VR and its rapidly increasing features, older persons could benefit from this emerging technology.

V. M. M. Anlacan, A. C. F. Panganiban and R. D. G. Jamora—These authors contributed equally to this work.

Keywords: Virtual reality (VR) · Persons living with dementia (PLDs) · Behavioral and psychological symptoms of dementia (BPSD) · Gamification · Personalization · Virtual environment design

1 Introduction

Dementia is characterized by an unusual progressive decline in cognition [17] that affects a person's autonomy in completing activities of daily living [6]. In the Philippines, dementia has an estimated prevalence of 10.6%, with 85.1% likely due to Alzheimer's disease (AD) - the most common form of dementia [8]. Commonly, persons living with dementia (PLDs) also experience changes in mood, behavior, emotional control, or motivation, collectively identified as behavioral and psychological symptoms of dementia (BPSD). BPSD tends to fluctuate and worsen as dementia progresses [17]. Inadequate management of BPSD may cause poor health outcomes for both the patient and their caregivers [11]. While pharmacological interventions are available, the effects of these medications are modest at best. Moreover, the intervention is limited due to potential side effects. Thus, there is a necessity to explore alternative, non-pharmacological interventions for managing BPSD [4].

In recent studies, immersive technologies have rapidly gained interest as one of the tools aiding the technological revolution in healthcare [1]. Immersive Virtual reality (VR) has been explored as an intervention for several clinical conditions. Some of these conditions are pain and anxiety [9, 14, 16], burns [7], phobias [15], and neurocognitive diseases [13]. Moreover, the inspirational affectation brought about by immersive VR [10] has led researchers to consider it for use among individuals with impaired memory, such as PLDs.

Previous works [2, 3] have explored utilizing immersive VR for managing BPSD among PLDs. Throughout these studies, the researchers have consistently collaborated with Philippine professionals and domain experts representing the fields of neurology, internal medicine, physiatry, nursing, anthropology, graphic design, game design, and software engineering for guidance and evaluation. With the initial 2022 study [3], the researchers have gathered requirements and identified constraints in administering BPSD therapy. The researchers have then designed and developed an initial prototype around it and acquired expert insights regarding its initial design and activities. Following this, the researchers have further improved the VR prototype in the recent 2023 study [2] by implementing additional features, addressing identified problems, and refining the virtual environment to the advantage of the target population. Sentiments acquired from domain experts regarding the improved VR prototype suggest its acceptability and acknowledgment of its potential for managing BPSD among PLDs in the Philippines.

In this paper, the researchers expand the 2023 study [2] by further refining and enhancing the VR prototype with concepts and features highly appreciated by domain experts. This is to further improve the effectiveness and usability of the VR application in preparation for a potential clinical evaluation. Throughout this paper, the researchers have expounded ideas and techniques for improving VR features which could serve as a guide or blueprint for future studies on designing VR applications suitable for PLDs.

The researchers have structured this paper into five distinct sections. The initial section serves as an introduction by providing an overview of the study and its context. The second section then establishes the foundation of the research by examining related studies in the literature. Through the third section, the researchers have presented the final refinements on the VR application for clinical evaluation. This section is then followed by a comprehensive discussion in the fourth section, regarding the refinements and their implications. Finally, the fifth and final section serves as the conclusion, summarizing the essential findings and implications of the VR intervention for BPSD therapy.

2 Review of Related Literature

Highlighting techniques utilized by applications or systems in recent literature, Martinho et al. [12] examined strategies that enhance well-being and quality of life among older persons. They observed that most applications used combinations of game design elements. For applications designed for training sessions, the combination of feedback, progression, time constraints, and score game design elements was common since these design elements provide effective and real-time performance indicators. Alternatively, applications designed to enhance relaxed gameplay utilized a combination of feedback, progression elements, a reward system, and social interaction. Rather than using time constraints or a score tracker that might make the experience competitive, entertaining features to enhance individual and collective gameplay could be incorporated into game applications.

Moreover, Martinho et al. [12] also elaborated on the challenges of recent game applications designed for older individuals. They emphasized that many studies failed to acknowledge the diverse living environments in which users may reside. As these users age, they became more vulnerable and have increasingly specific needs. Thus, game application development should consider these potential needs to ensure their usability and effectiveness for older persons.

Considering the specific needs of older individuals, the researchers, through previous works [3], explored utilizing immersive VR for managing BPSD among PLD living in Manila, Philippines. In the initial 2022 study [2,3], the researchers identified the requirements and constraints for implementing a BPSD therapy using immersive VR. Building upon these findings and drawing from design strategies employed in VR studies documented in the literature, the researchers developed the initial prototype of a VR game application. Using this VR prototype as a foundation for iterative development, the researchers conducted alpha testing and a focus group discussion (FGD) with domain experts. The results of the FGD provided profound insights and recommendations on the design and architecture of the VR prototype to enhance its potential usability and acceptability for older individuals.

Incorporating the inspiration and recommendations derived from the initial 2022 study [3], the researchers made significant improvements to the VR prototype in their subsequent study [2]. These improvements entailed implementing additional features, resolving identified issues, and refining the virtual environment. Noteworthy enhancements incorporated into the improved VR prototype encompassed the following key aspects:

- *Virtual Companion and Observation or Control Module.* The enhanced VR prototype introduced a virtual companion with the visual representation of a child. To ensure dynamic and engaging interactions, a trained therapist provided real-time piloting and voice acting for the companion. This virtual companion served as a guide, offering directions, engaging in spontaneous conversations, and performing predefined animations using the observation or control module, enhancing the immersive experience for the participants.
- *Initiator.* The initiator component was used as an introduction to the VR user interface. It served as a tutorial environment where users could practice interacting with objects and navigating within the virtual space before engaging in the actual VR game. It provided a structured and guided experience, familiarizing users with the essential controls, functionalities, and movements required for seamless participation in the VR application.
- *Hand Tracking and Gestures.* Hand tracking refers to the real-time tracking and mapping of a user's hand movements in the virtual environment. This innovative feature empowered participants to engage with virtual objects solely through their physical hands. By accurately capturing and translating hand motions into the virtual world, users seamlessly interacted with virtual objects, enhancing the immersive and intuitive nature of the VR experience.

The researchers then again conducted alpha testing and a focus group discussion (FGD) among domain experts. The sentiments from FGD indicated a positive reception toward the overall design of the VR prototype. Participants appreciated that the environment and objects within the virtual setting reflected Filipino and old-fashioned aesthetics. These deliberate design choices fostered a cohesive environment and instilled a sense of familiarity. The domain experts showcased a level of acceptability and recognition for the VR prototype's potential in managing BPSD among PLDs in the Philippines.

Previous research also explored the development of tools to facilitate the design of virtual environments (VEs) based on real-world settings. One such tool was the BENOGO Place probe developed by Benyon et al. [5]. The place probe aimed to capture the essence of a real-world location (sense of place) and translate it into a form that developers could replicate in the virtual world. Results of the study indicated that the virtual environment created with the place probe yielded comparable experiences for participants in contrast to the original real-world location. This suggests that developers can leverage the insights provided by the place probe to design more immersive and convincing virtual environments.

3 VR Therapy Game Application

The VR game prototype presented in this paper incorporates improvements based on previous publications [2,3]. These improvements were implemented to enhance the efficacy and usability of the VR application to prepare for a potential clinical evaluation.

The improved VR prototype continued to offer an experience centered around visiting familiar or historical locations, fostering relaxation, and invoking pleasant memories within the simulated environment and activities.

3.1 Virtual Companion and Observation/Control Module

In line with previous work [2], the VR prototype featured a virtual companion piloted by a trained therapist. The companion served as a guide, offering directions, engaging in spontaneous conversations, and performing predefined animations using the observation or control module, enhancing the immersive experience for the participants. Other features still included in the observation module were: the guide for the flow of the session, a companion animation wheel, a timer, a view of the participant in real-time, and the view of the participant in the virtual environment. The interface of the Observation/Control Module as viewed by the therapist is shown in Fig. 1.

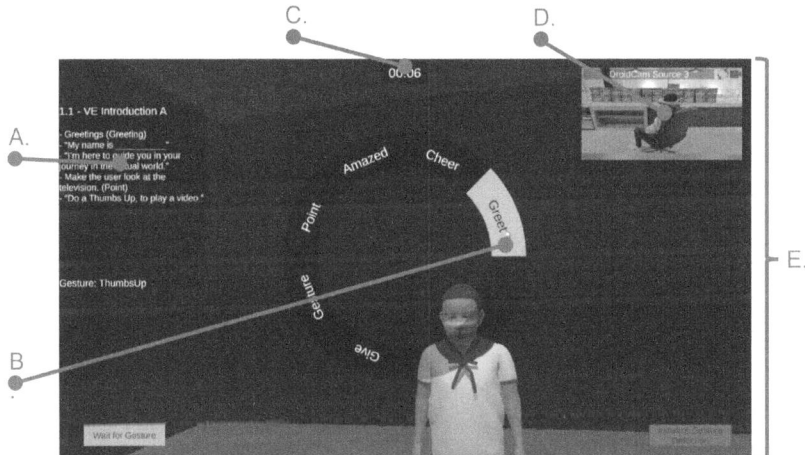

Fig. 1. Observation Module (as viewed by the therapist) [2]. (A) Guide for the flow of the session, (B) companion animation wheel, (C) timer, (D) view of the participant in real-time, (E) participant's view of the VE without the module interface A to D, and (F) the boy in white is the virtual companion.

Recognizing the need for diversity, an option of a girl companion model was introduced at the beginning of the therapy session to represent female therapists. The companion models are showcased in Fig. 2. Furthermore, the improved prototype provided the therapist with additional capabilities through the observation module. With the enhanced functionality, the therapist could redo, stop, and pause the virtual activities or the therapy session itself. This allowed for proactive measures to address unforeseen adverse events or bugs. The added flexibility empowered the therapist to ensure a smoother and safer experience for the participants, enabling prompt intervention if needed.

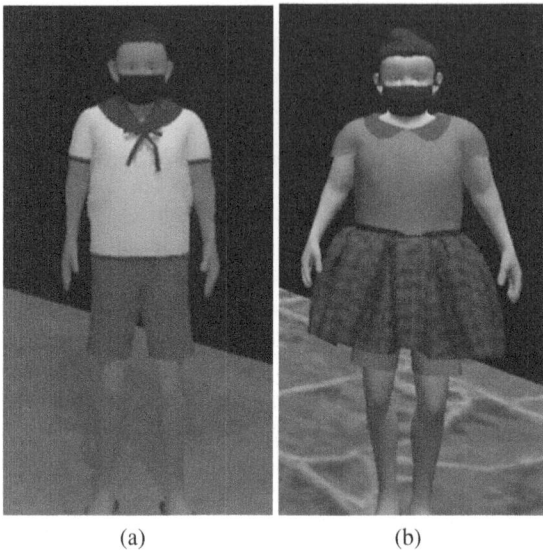

Fig. 2. Models of the virtual companion: (a) boy companion model and (b) girl companion model. The therapist could choose their prefered model at the start of the session.

3.2 Initiator

The initiator served as a tutorial environment where users could practice interacting with objects and navigating within the virtual space before engaging in the actual VR game. In previous work [2], it helped familiarize users with the essential controls, functionalities, and movements required for seamless participation in the VR application. Activities included in the initiator are displayed in Fig. 3.

To further enhance the overall user experience, the researchers made minor modifications to the initiator component. These adjustments encompassed two key factors. Firstly, audio feedback was incorporated into the activities within the initiator to improve object interaction. Secondly, the positions of objects in the user's hands were appropriately adjusted to facilitate a more realistic and convincing object manipulation. These modifications aimed to refine the initiator's functionality and design, ultimately contributing to a more engaging user experience.

3.3 Hand Tracking and Gestures

Hand tracking refers to the real-time tracking and mapping of a user's hand movements in the virtual environment as demonstrated in Fig. 4. This advanced capability enables participants to interact with virtual objects exclusively using their physical hands. In this version of the VR prototype, the hand-tracking feature continued to be implemented for natural interaction between users and the virtual world.

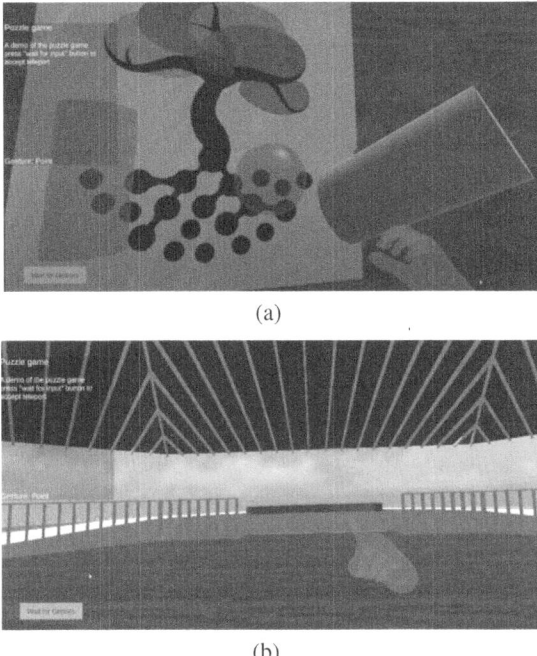

(a)

(b)

Fig. 3. Activities in the Initiator: (a) participant interacting with virtual objects and matching their shapes and (b) participant initiating teleportation using the pointing hand gesture.

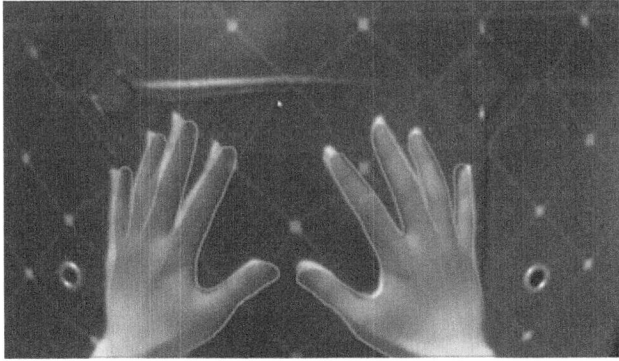

Fig. 4. Hand-tracking demonstration.

3.4 Multiple Virtual Environments

In previous works [2,3], the Rizal Park virtual environment (VE) served as the primary setting for participants to engage in recreational activities and freely explore with the therapist. The VE's structure incorporated a 360-degree image of Rizal Park as the background, while virtual objects were generated to represent key landmarks and structures within the park. The Place Probe from [5] was utilized to capture the essence of the park and determine these key landmarks and structures. The resulting VE depicted an open space that closely mirrored the visual and auditory ambiance of the actual Rizal Park in Manila, Philippines. Screenshots of the virtual Rizal Park and the actual Rizal Park located in Manila, Philippines are displayed in Fig. 5.

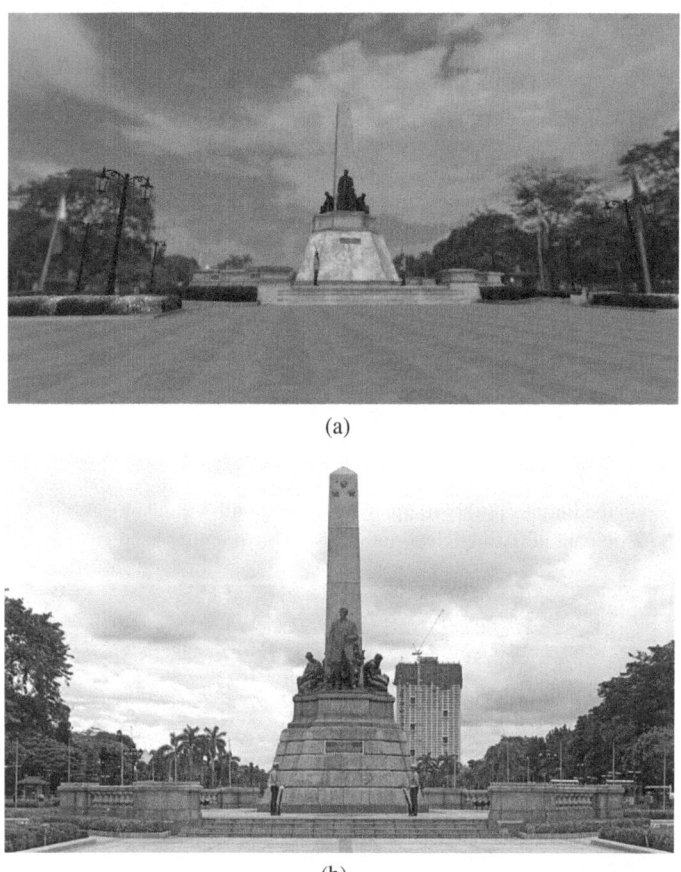

(a)

(b)

Fig. 5. Screenshot of (a) the virtual Rizal Park and (b) the Rizal Park located at Manila, Philippines.

Leveraging these concepts of VE construction, the researchers developed two additional VEs: the Palawan VE and the Church VE. The Palawan VE drew inspiration from a cliffside location in Palawan, Philippines, accentuating nature-oriented characteristics that differed from the urban ambiance of the classical Rizal Park VE. Alongside the Palawan VE, the researchers also generated the Church VE that depicts old Roman Catholic churches scattered across the Philippines. The primary inspiration for this VE was the Barosoain church located in Malolos, Bulacan. These new virtual environments

(VEs) provided diverse surroundings to explore and engage in that could enhance the overall richness and depth of the immersive experiences for the participants.

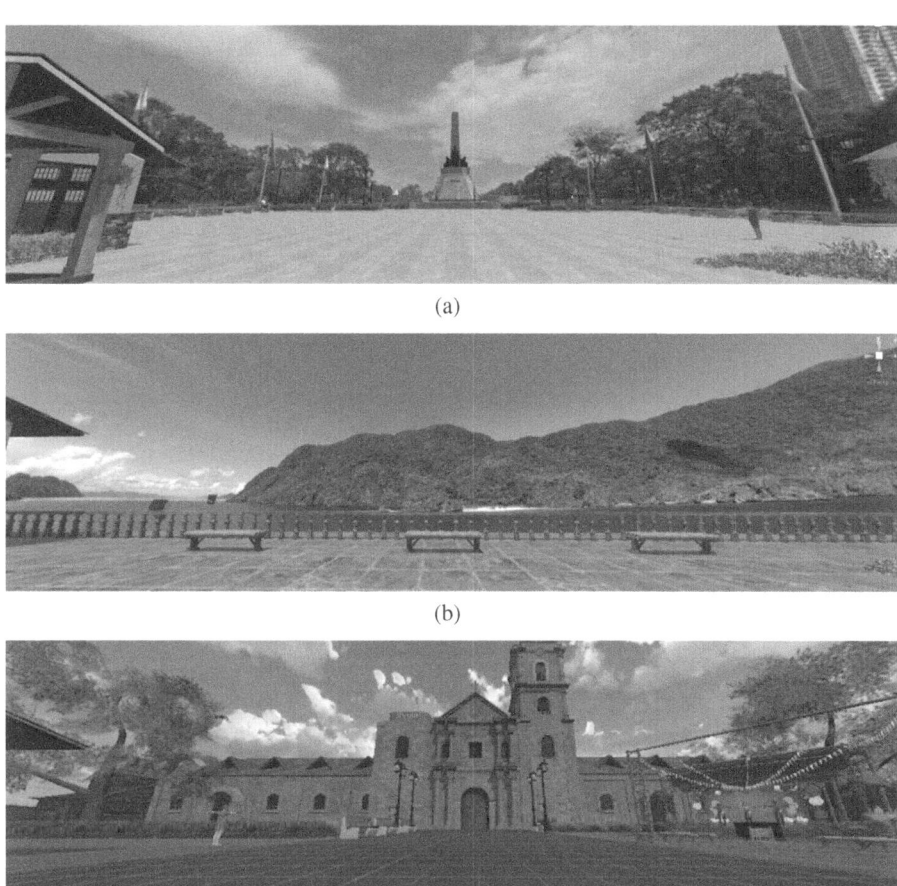

Fig. 6. Developed virtual environments: (a) the virtual Rizal Park, (b) the virtual cliffside located at Palawan, Philippines, and (c) virtual church inspired by the Barosoain church located in Malolos, Bulacan.

3.5 Virtual Activities

The VR application incorporated various recreational activities for participants to engage in. The initial prototype [3] featured two primary activities: Avatar Customization and Painting activity. In the Avatar Customization room, users had the opportunity to decorate their virtual avatars (virtual representations of themselves in the virtual environment) with clothing inspired by traditional Filipino dresses and accessories. This room aimed to foster a stronger connection between the user and their avatar by allowing them to personalize and customize its appearance according to their preferences. The second activity, inspired by art therapy, was the Painting activity. Users were able to paint or add colors to a collection of initially colorless (white) flowers. This activity offered freedom to express their creativity and preferences through artistic expression.

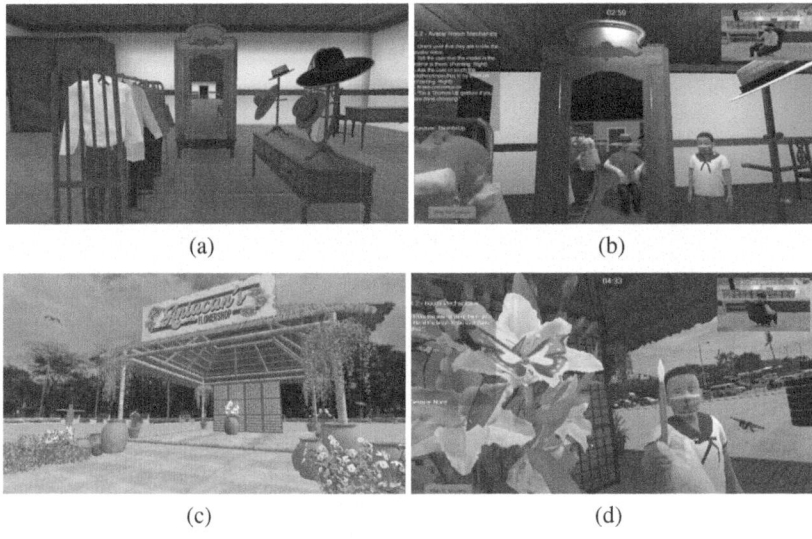

Fig. 7. (a) Avatar Customization Room, (b) participant customizing their avatar, (c) Painting Booth, and (d) companion giving the participant a paintbrush to paint the flowers.

In the second prototype [2], the researchers made significant improvements to the activities introduced in the initial prototype by enhancing usability and overall user experience based on the result of the 2022 study [3]. Additionally, a new activity called the Puzzle activity was included. This activity drew inspiration from occupational therapy practices. In the Puzzle activity, users were tasked with assembling various parts of

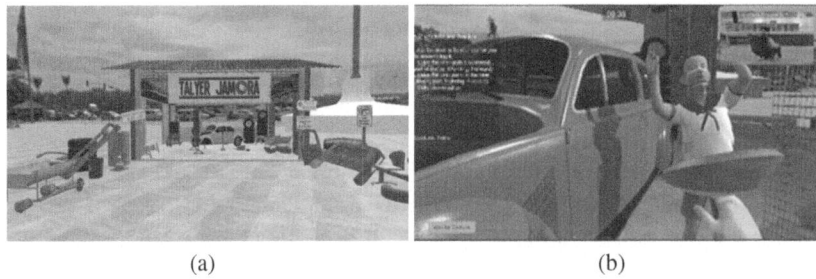

Fig. 8. (a) Puzzle Booth and (b) participant assembling the car.

a car. The purpose of this activity was to engage and challenge the participant's cognitive abilities within the virtual environment.

In this study, the researchers made significant improvements to the introduced activities based on the findings of the 2023 study [2] by further enhancing usability and overall user experience. Additionally, a new activity called the Singing activity was included. This activity drew inspiration from music therapy practices. The Singing activity added a musical element to the VR experience. In this activity, participants were invited to take part in a mini-concert featuring an old Filipino song. The activity aimed to provide relaxation and enjoyment to the participants while also offering them the opportunity to participate using a virtual musical instrument.

During each iteration of the VR application, significant improvements were made to enhance the overall user experience by focusing on relaxation and enjoyment within the VR environment. Furthermore, new activities were introduced, representing different therapy practices to offer variation and cater to a wider range of potential users. All activities incorporated common game elements, such as visual and auditory feedback, progression elements, a rewarding system, and social interaction with the therapist-companion. These elements were in line with the recommendations of Martinho et al. [12] in providing relaxed gameplay and enhanced overall user experience.

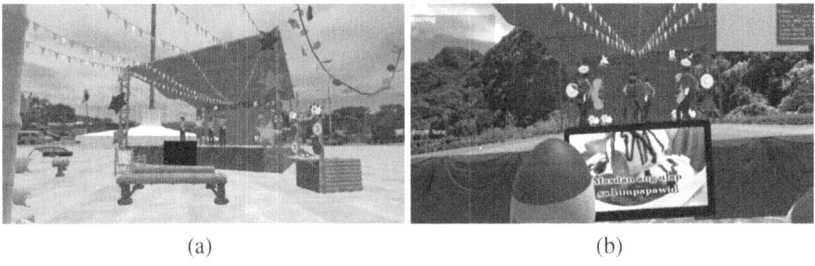

(a) (b)

Fig. 9. (a) Singing Booth and (b) participant enjoying the mini-concert with their maracas.

3.6 VR Testing Setup and Flow

Similar to previous works [2,3], the testing setup recommended for the VR application would include a dedicated "play area" of $9\,\text{m}^2\,(3\,\text{m} \times 3\,\text{m})$ allocated for the participant and a workstation for the VR therapist and the experiment observer (researcher). This setup would allow comfortable and unobstructed movement for the participant while inside the virtual environment. Moreover, the researchers still recommended that the participant remain seated throughout the experiment for their safety. Figure 10 offers an overview of the testing setup.

The experiment would start after the user successfully put on the VR HMD and earphones with the assistance of the researchers, and ended upon the participant's completion of all activities and the removal of the HMD. An overview of the flow of activities in the VR Game prototype is shown in Fig. 11.

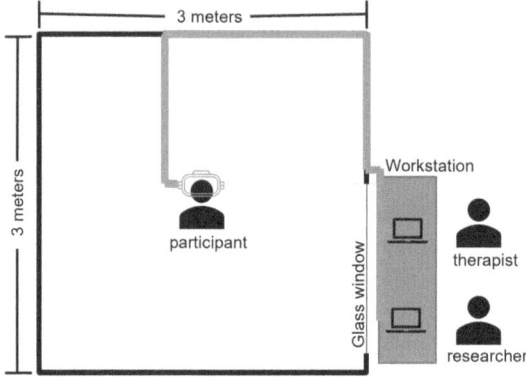

Fig. 10. Overview of the recommended testing setup [2].

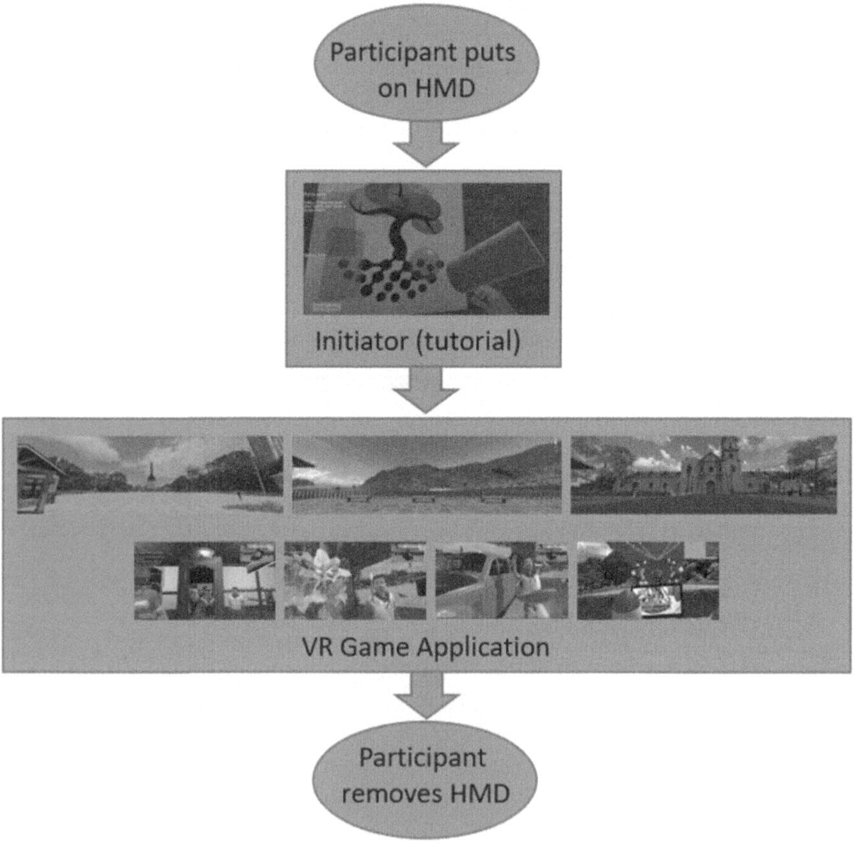

Fig. 11. Flow of the VR session.

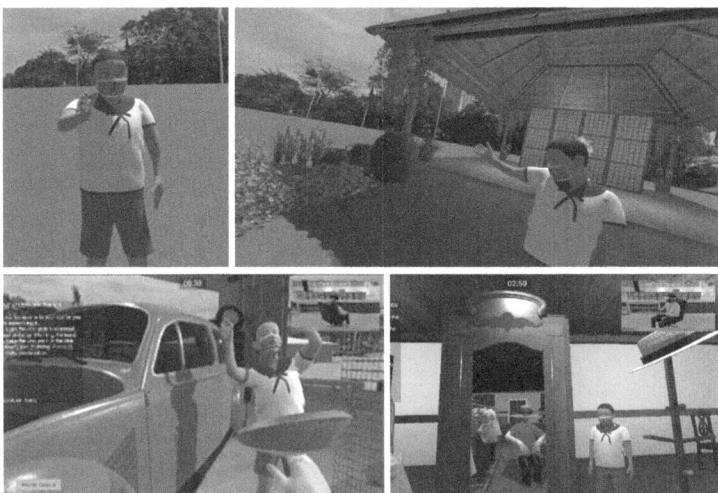

Fig. 12. The virtual companion guiding and interacting with the participant throughout the VR experience.

4 Discussion

4.1 Development Notes

During each iteration of the VR prototype, the researchers maintained ongoing communication with domain experts to create VR experiences that could serve as an alternative, non-pharmacological intervention for managing BPSD. The domain experts played a vital role in providing valuable insights regarding the VR application. Their input was crucial in identifying unknown problems and unanticipated implications of the intervention throughout each iteration. Future iterations would continue to follow similar approaches and procedures to ensure the quality and relevance of the VR application.

In terms of the VR experience, the addition of a VR therapist as a companion had a remarkable impact on creating a sense of connection for the users within the VR environment. The VR therapist, playing the role of a guide and a genuine companion, offered the needed social interaction recommended by Martinho et al. [12]. Participants visually enjoyed the experience more when they had someone to share the moment with, as observed in the transition from the initial prototype without a therapist to the second prototype with the therapist-companion. Furthermore, interactions could be further leveraged by incorporating structured conversation prompts from the therapist - maximizing the therapeutic potential of the VR experience.

The initiator served as an important component in introducing participants to the virtual world. Even though immersive VR mimics real-life interactions, the concept of 360-degree viewing and navigating within virtual environments could be foreign to many individuals. With the assistance of the therapist-companion, the initiator played a significant role in easing the transition into this new technological experience. It was recommended that future studies also incorporate an initiator in their VR applications

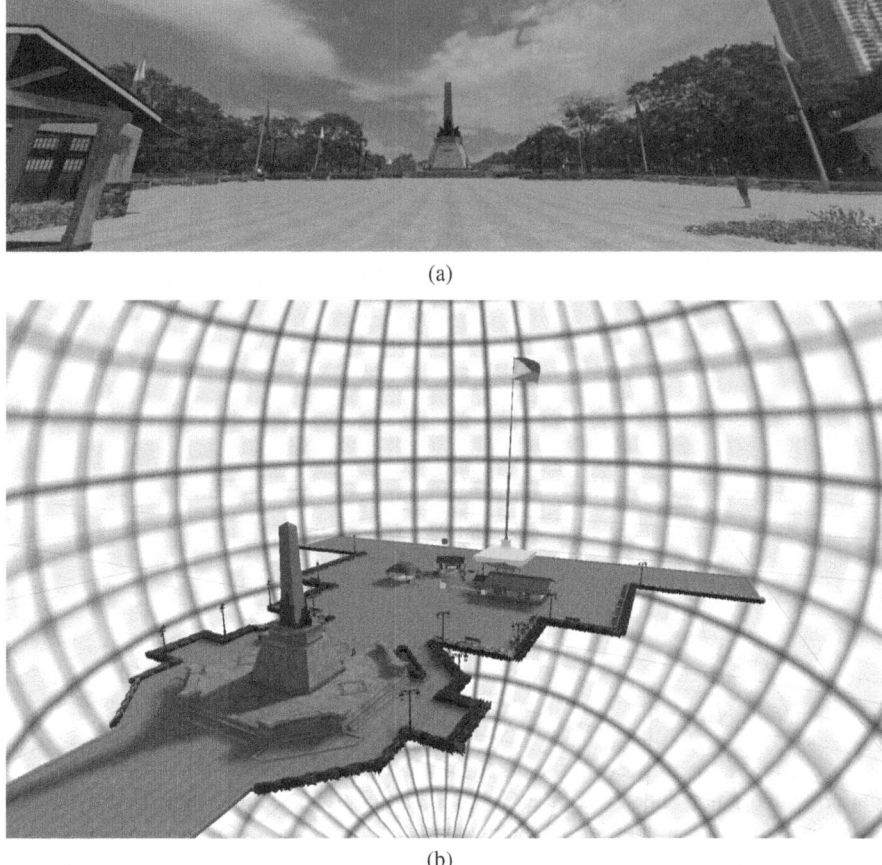

Fig. 13. (a) virtual Rizal Park as viewed by the participants in the HMD and (b) structure of the virtual Rizal Park without the 360-degree background image of the actual Rizal Park.

to assist participants, regardless of their technological background, in taking their initial steps into immersive virtual reality.

By harnessing the capabilities of virtual reality, a personalized and controlled virtual environment might be simulated and designed to the advantage of the target population. The researchers developed a systematic strategy, inspired by the Place Probe of Benyon et al. [5], to capture the essence of real-world locations and replicate them within the virtual world. This approach allowed for the creation of various virtual environments tailored to the preferences of the target population, thereby enhancing the personalization of the VR application. Additionally, activities could be integrated seamlessly into these environments based on the specifications of therapists or therapy practices. The study recommended incorporating game elements, as identified by Martinho et al. [12], that align with the goals of their VR application. However, the researchers also

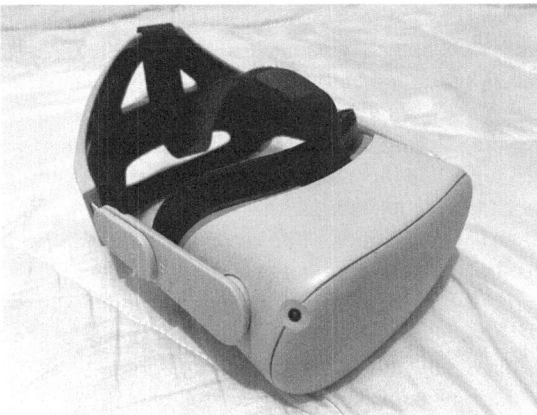

Fig. 14. The Oculus Quest 2 (Meta Quest 2) head-mounted display.

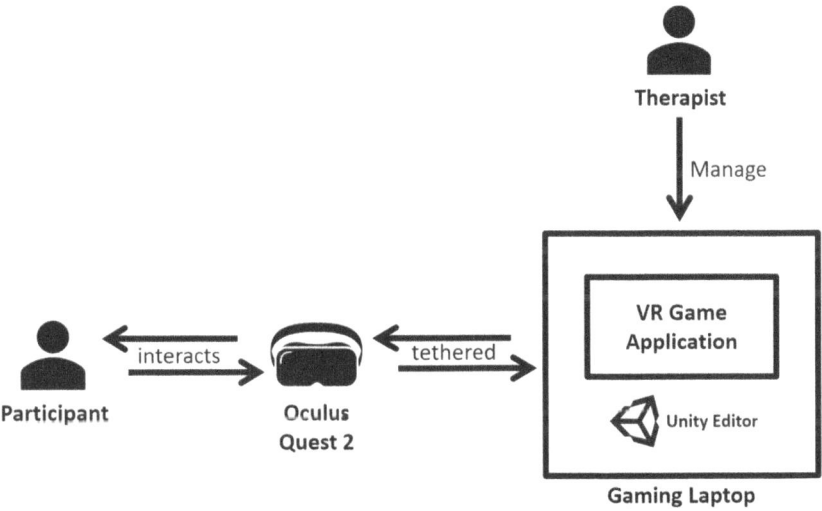

Fig. 15. Game architecture for the experiment to optimize quality and performance of the VR application. participant interacts with the Oculus Quest 2 VR HMD to navigate the VR application. The VR HMD is tethered to a powerful gaming laptop which runs the VR application using the Unity Editor.

encouraged exploring different combinations of identified game elements to determine the most appropriate approach for achieving their therapeutic objectives.

4.2 Implications and Limitations

The primary objective of the VR application was to offer an immersive experience that promotes relaxation and evokes pleasant memories. The VR application accomplished this by offering a diverse range of virtual environments to explore and various recreational activities to engage in. However, the researchers acknowledged the possibility of participants becoming accustomed to the activities over repeated sessions. To address this concern in future iterations, the researchers planned to introduce variations in the elements of each activity. This would ensure participants encounter something new and refreshing during each session. By incorporating these variations, the researchers expected to sustain the interest and engagement of participants.

Regarding the technical requirements, the VR application was developed using the Unity game engine and was designed to be compatible with the Meta (Oculus) Quest 2 head-mounted display (HMD). The native features of Meta Quest 2, such as hand-tracking, played a crucial role in enhancing the user-friendliness of the VR application. However, the researchers observed that the computing power of the HMD was insufficient to ensure a consistently smooth experience. Minor lags and performance drops were observed in certain parts of the virtual environment. These anomalies should be taken into consideration as they can contribute to the occurrence of VR simulator sickness - impacting the overall user experience. Addressing these issues and optimizing performance was important to provide users with a seamless and enjoyable VR experience.

In order to ensure consistent and optimal quality and performance during the Alpha testing in the 2023 study [2], the researchers employed a tethered setup for the Meta Quest HMD. They connected the VR headset to a gaming laptop (Nitro AN515-45, AMD Ryzen 7 5800H, 16 GB RAM, Windows 11 64-bit) to offload the heavy processing and rendering tasks to the more powerful laptop. Through this configuration, the VR HMD was only displaying the virtual environment and acquiring user interaction through its sensors. However, one drawback of this setup was the restriction of motion due to the tethered connection between the VR HMD and the laptop.

5 Conclusion

In conclusion, this paper presented the refined and enhanced VR therapy game application designed for managing BPSDs among PLDs in the Philippines. Building upon previous works, the improvements included the refinement of the virtual companion, enhancements to the observation/control module, the development of different virtual environments, and the addition of a new recreational activity. These refinements aimed to improve the effectiveness, usability, and overall user experience in preparation for potential clinical evaluation.

The VR therapy game application could offer a promising non-pharmacological intervention for managing BPSD - addressing the limitations of pharmacological treatments and providing a more personalized and engaging approach to dementia care. Future studies could build upon the ideas and techniques presented in this paper for refining and expanding their respective VR therapy game application. Continued collaboration with healthcare professionals, domain experts, and end-users would be crucial in ensuring the applicability, acceptability, and effectiveness of this innovative intervention. With the versatility of VR and its rapidly increasing features for usability, older persons could benefit from this emerging technology.

Acknowledgments. The authors of this paper would like to thank the Republic of the Philippines Department of Science and Technology Philippine Council for Health Research and Development and the University of the Philippines - Manila (Reference Number: RGAO-2018-0573-01) for funding this research.

References

1. Andringa, G., et al.: Feasibility of virtual reality in elderly with dementia. In: Brankaert, R., IJsselsteijn, W. (eds.) D-Lab 2019. CCIS, vol. 1117, pp. 146–149. Springer, Cham (2019). https://doi.org/10.1007/978-3-030-33540-3_14
2. Anlacan, V., et al.: Analysis of virtual reality therapy game prototype for persons living with dementia in the Philippines. In: Proceedings of the 16th International Joint Conference on Biomedical Engineering Systems and Technologies - HEALTHINF, pp. 144–154. INSTICC, SciTePress (2023). https://doi.org/10.5220/0011686900003414
3. Anlacan, V.M.M., et al.: Application design for a virtual reality therapy game for patients with behavioral and psychological symptoms of dementia. In: Krouska, A., Troussas, C., Caro, J. (eds.) NiDS 2022. LNNS, vol. 556, pp. 149–160. Springer, Cham (2022). https://doi.org/10.1007/978-3-031-17601-2_15
4. Appel, L., et al.: Administering virtual reality therapy to manage behavioral and psychological symptoms in patients with dementia admitted to an acute care hospital: results of a pilot study. JMIR Formative Res. **5**(2), e22406 (2021)
5. Benyon, D., Smyth, M., O'Neill, S., McCall, R., Carroll, F.: The place probe: exploring a sense of place in real and virtual environments. Presence Teleoper. Virtual Environ. **15**(6), 668–687 (2006)
6. Chertkow, H., Feldman, H.H., Jacova, C., Massoud, F.: Definitions of dementia and predementia states in Alzheimer's disease and vascular cognitive impairment: consensus from the Canadian conference on diagnosis of dementia. Alzheimer's Res. Therapy **5**(1), 1–8 (2013)
7. Czech, O., Wrzeciono, A., Baťalík, B., Szczepańska-Gieracha, S.G., Malicka, I., Rutkowski, S.: Virtual reality intervention as a support method during wound care and rehabilitation after burns: a systematic review and meta-analysis. Complement. Ther. Med. 102837 (2022)
8. Dominguez, J., de Guzman, F., Reandelar, M., Jr., Thi Phung, T.K., et al.: Prevalence of dementia and associated risk factors: a population-based study in the Philippines. J. Alzheimers Dis. **63**(3), 1065–1073 (2018)
9. Eijlers, R., et al.: Meta-analysis: systematic review and meta-analysis of virtual reality in pediatrics: effects on pain and anxiety. Anesth. Analg. **129**(5), 1344 (2019)
10. Huntsman, M.: How a virtual reality forest helps Alzheimer's patients. Alzheimers.net (2014). https://tinyurl.com/5xxtykpv. https://www.alzheimers.net/how-a-virtual-reality-forest-helps-alzheimers-patients
11. Kales, H.C., Gitlin, L.N., Lyketsos, C.G.: Assessment and management of behavioral and psychological symptoms of dementia. BMJ **350** (2015)
12. Martinho, D., Carneiro, J., Corchado, J.M., Marreiros, G.: A systematic review of gamification techniques applied to elderly care. Artif. Intell. Rev. **53**(7), 4863–4901 (2020)
13. Moreno, A., Wall, K.J., Thangavelu, K., Craven, L., Ward, E., Dissanayaka, N.N.: A systematic review of the use of virtual reality and its effects on cognition in individuals with neurocognitive disorders. Alzheimer's Dementia Transl. Res. Clin. Interv. **5**, 834–850 (2019)
14. Pourmand, A., Davis, S., Marchak, A., Whiteside, T., Sikka, N.: Virtual reality as a clinical tool for pain management. Curr. Pain Headache Rep. **22**(8), 1–6 (2018)

15. Wechsler, T.F., Kümpers, F., Mühlberger, A.: Inferiority or even superiority of virtual reality exposure therapy in phobias?-a systematic review and quantitative meta-analysis on randomized controlled trials specifically comparing the efficacy of virtual reality exposure to gold standard in vivo exposure in agoraphobia, specific phobia, and social phobia. Front. Psychol. 1758 (2019)
16. Wittkopf, P.G., Lloyd, D.M., Coe, O., Yacoobali, S., Billington, J.: The effect of interactive virtual reality on pain perception: a systematic review of clinical studies. Disabil. Rehabil. **42**(26), 3722–3733 (2020)
17. World-Health-Organization: Dementia (2022). who.int. https://www.who.int/news-room/fact-sheets/detail/dementia

The Impact of Feature Selection on Balancing, Based on Diabetes Data

Diogo Machado[1,3], Vítor Santos Costa[2,3(✉)], and Pedro Brandão[1,3(✉)]

[1] Instituto de Telecomunicações, Aveiro, Portugal
[2] INESC-TEC, Porto, Portugal
vsc@dcc.fc.up.pt
[3] Faculdade de Ciências da Universidade do Porto, Porto, Portugal
{dmachado,pbrandao}@dcc.fc.up.pt

Abstract. Diabetes management data is composed of diverse factors and glycaemia indicators. Glycaemia predictive models tend to focus solely on glycaemia values. A comprehensive understanding of diabetes management requires the consideration of several aspects of diabetes management, beyond glycaemia. However, the inclusion of every aspect of diabetes management can create an overly high-dimensional data set. Excessive feature spaces increase computational complexity and may introduce over-fitting. Additionally, the inclusion of inconsequential features introduces noise that hinders a model's performance. Feature importance is a process that evaluates a feature's value, and can be used to identify optimal feature sub-sets. Depending on the context, multiple methods can be used. The drop feature method, in the literature, is considered to be the best approach to evaluate individual feature importance. To reach an optimal set, the best approach is branch and bound, albeit its heavy computational cost. This overhead can be addressed through a trade-off between the feature set's optimisation level and the process' computational feasibility. The improvement of the feature space has implications on the effectiveness of data balancing approaches. Whilst, in this study, the observed impact was not substantial, it warrants the need to reconsider the balancing approach given a superior feature space.

Keywords: Diabetes · Data-mining · Feature importance · Data imbalance

1 Introduction

Diabetes is a chronic disease characterised by high blood glucose levels, resultant of the patient's deficiency in insulin action, production or both. It is calculated that 463 million people around the world in 2019 suffered from diabetes. This number is projected to reach 700 million by 2045 [10]. Diabetes management aims at improving the patient's life quality and expectancy through a strict glycaemia supervision. It is vital for patients to maintain glucose levels within a normal range, and minimise episodes of hyperglycaemia (abnormally high glycaemia levels) or hypoglycaemia (abnormally low glycaemia levels), which can be life-threatening. In the long term, repeated exposure to hyperglycaemia damages the blood vessels, and may lead to blindness, heart problems, increased risk of having a stroke, among other serious health issues. Extreme occurrences of hyperglycaemia or hypoglycaemia may result in a comatose state, and even death [23,29,30].

The correct management of diabetes entails frequent glycaemia testing, and a conscious balance of meals and insulin. Additionally, patients must consider daily physical efforts, or exercise, illness, stress, among other factors that may influence glycaemia values. The patient's data contains knowledge essential to understand the intricacies that lead to occurrences of hypo or hyperglycaemia. Insight on the lead causes of these occurrences allows patients to improve their diabetes management.

Data mining is a process that analyses and extracts knowledge from a data set [25]. It is present, with positive results, in many health-domains such as liver diseases, cardiovascular diseases, cancer, and diabetes [31]. In the context of diabetes, data mining can be used to predict, and potentially prevent, hypo and hyperglycaemia events. Given the severity of these occurrences, most diabetic patients attempt, to the best of their ability, to stay within a glycaemia range considered normal. Therefore, diabetes management-based data sets are imbalanced, as most glycaemia observations will be normal. This is often the case in health related data sets [16]. Data imbalances cause bias towards the majority class [16], and may induce misleading conclusions. The use of data balancing methods can minimise these discrepancies. The study by Machado et al. [19] concluded that, for diabetes management-based data, the use of the balancing methodologies SMOTE and ENN is preferred. The success of under-sampling proves that, in data mining, "more" is not always an indicator of "better".

Analogously, the consideration of every aspect of a data set may hinder the model's performance. Features represent different data characteristics, hence, intuitively, more features should imply a deeper knowledge of the target, and consequently improve the model's performance. In reality, high-dimensional data poses a set number of challenges beyond its heavy computational costs. First, redundant or less relevant features may act as a source of noise. Additionally, a high number of dimensions may lead to data sparsity, and inhibit the model's performance [17]: the "curse of dimensionality". These data sets can also lead to over-fitting [12,17,35]. Therefore, attaining an optimal feature set should be considered essential.

A prior work by Machado et al. [19] studied the impact of different balancing methods on diabetes-based data. The focus of this work was purely on performance enhancements through balancing, therefore the data sets possessed their full feature space. This work's objective is to understand the impact of feature importance on the balancing method's performance. Additionally, we verify whether Machado et al. [19]'s results on the best balancing methods hold for an optimal feature set.

In Sect. 2 we will describe the methods used for the evaluation of feature importance, characterise the data-set used for the experiments, and motivate the need for re-evaluating the data balancing methods. Section 3 shows and analyses the feature importance evaluation. In Sect. 4 we analyse the impact of using the best feature set on the choice of balancing methods. Finally, Sect. 5 describes our main conclusions and the importance of the balancing approach chosen.

2 Methodology

The study of feature importance allows the pruning of inconsequential features, enhances predictive accuracy, improves comprehensibility and reduces model execution time [15, 18]. Additionally, through feature importance, it is possible to assert the main contributors to certain aspects of the target variable. In this work's context, the high relevance of a certain feature set may be indicative of a diabetes management issue that is causing hypo or hyperglycaemia.

Diabetic patients are seen as unique in their innate characteristics, and it is feasible that different patients' data will favour features differently. The variance in feature importance can be connected to multiple factors, including the lack of records by patients.

The two main approaches to the study of feature importance are: **(i)** the individual feature study; **(ii)** the search for the optimal feature set, in the data set's feature space. Each approach possesses multiple processes, each with different complexities and perceived accuracy.

2.1 Individual Feature Importance

Individual feature importance focuses on calculating the individual contribution of each feature to a model's performance. The simplest form of feature importance, only computable through tree-based models, is Mean Decrease Impurity (MDI), also known as Gini importance. This method evaluates the sum of all the decreases in impurity in a split, by a given feature, normalised by the number of trees. Although fast, a known issue of this metric is its bias towards categorical variables with higher representation [6, 27, 32].

Another common approach, but more complex, is the Mean Decrease Accuracy (MDA), also known as permutation importance. MDA measures feature importance by analysing the model's decrease in performance when the values of a feature are disarranged. A known problem with this metric is its tendency to overestimate correlated predictor variables [27, 32].

Although commonly used methods, MDI and MDA, are not true representations of feature importance [33]. To achieve a value closest to the real importance, other, more computationally demanding methods, have to be used.

In terms of individual feature importance, the drop feature method is to be preferred [33]. This method evaluates the difference in performance, for each feature, that occurs when a feature is "dropped". The process begins with the computation of the baseline, a metric that represents the performance of the data set with its full feature space. Subsequently, for each feature, it is calculated the performance of the data set with the full feature set, excepting the feature to be evaluated. The difference between the baseline and the value of the performance without the feature depicts how important the feature is. While more accurate, this method is more computationally demanding, as it requires the training and testing of a model multiple times (one for each feature, plus the baseline) [33].

2.2 Optimal Feature Set Search

The optimal set selection method emphasises the relevance of group importance, in opposition to individual importance. In many situations, a feature's importance is not fully individual. Some features only reach their full potential when paired with other features. By determining an optimal feature set, it is possible to understand which features have a main role for a model, albeit it is not possible to grasp how much each feature contributes. Optimal feature search can be broadly divided in two processes: search organisation, and successor generation [15]. Molina et al. [22] consider the Evaluation measure as a third subset selection process.

Search Organisation. The search organisation consists of the different search strategies available to explore the feature space. Considering the number of possible subsets, it may not be feasible to search all the possible combinations of features. Sequential search is a type of search organisation that follows a greedy logic. At each step of this method all successors are evaluated, and one is chosen. Once a successor is chosen, the method will not backtrack. To be classified as a sequential search, the method must be of $O(n)$ complexity order. This method gives completeness, but does not guarantee the best feature set.

To ensure the best feature set through search organisation, exponential search is more appropriate. It is an exhaustive type of search that uses heuristics functions to reduce the number of possibilities within the search space. Branch and bound [24], and Beam search [7] are two examples of exponential searches. Another method that could qualify, given an admissible heuristic, is A^* [22].

Another option that can secure the optimal solution is Random search. This process introduces randomness to break the normal sequence of search, that prioritises local and sequential subsets. Another option is to create a fully random subset of features at each iteration, following the Las Vegas algorithm [2].

Successor Generation. The generation of successors is the process responsible for creating alternatives to the current hypothesis. The result of each iteration of this process is a new feature set to be evaluated. Five different types of operations can be performed to generate a new successor: forward, backward, compound, weighting, and random.

The Forward Process: begins with an empty optimal feature set, and adds, at each iteration, the best option available amidst the choices that have not been selected previously. The method ends when one of the following cases occur: all the available features have been selected; the optimal feature set's evaluation does not increase with further iterations; manual limiters are reached e.g. the set has reached a certain desired score.

The Backward Process: follows the inverse approach of the forward process. The process begins with a full feature set as the optimal solution. The features that are part of the current solution are removed and the set is evaluated. The feature that, when excluded, enhances the most the set's performance is removed. The process concludes when: no more features can be removed; if it is not possible to increase the set's performance by removing features; or by manual limiters.

The Compound Process: consists on applying a certain amount of consecutive forward processes and a second amount of backward processes. If the number of backward and forward processes is the same, the end result set will be the original set, meaning the process cannot further improve, thus the process is concluded. The choice between the number of forward and backward steps can be set manually, or determined according to the current "optimal set's" evaluation.

The Weighting Process: sets a different weight to each feature according to their importance. This is achieved by iterative sampling across the available subset space.

The Random Process: breaks the sequential nature of the previous methods. This process generates random subsets in terms of feature organisation and set-size.

2.3 Data Set Overview

The data set used to evaluate feature importance will be based on the one used by Machado et al. [19]. Instead of using both sets featured in this work, the analysis of feature importance will be focused solely on the data set derived from the Ohio data set [21], and not using the St. Louis data set [13]. Comparing both sets, the Ohio data set possesses a smaller patient pool. In terms of feature-space, the Ohio data set encompasses the full spectrum of features present in the St. Louis data set, whilst also incorporating sensor-based features absent in the St. Louis data set. As Continuous Glucose Monitor (CGM) devices become more common, patient's data will gravitate towards the feature typology present in the Ohio data set. Finger-prick-based data sets continue to be relevant, not only because many patients still do not use CGM, but also because they contain important data that may be used to uncover hypo and hyperglycaemia data [20].

In terms of features, the data set contains, in addition to the glycaemia designation that is the target feature, seven *sensor-based glycaemia* features, seven *finger-based glycaemia* features, three features representing *manual alterations to basal insulin*, one *existence of meal* feature, one *existence of insulin* feature, one *existence of exercise* feature, one *existence of effort* feature, the designation of the record's *day of the week*, and the designation of the record's *time of day*. The non-glycaemia-based features are associated with five time intervals: [T, T-30min], [T-30min, T-1 h], [T-1h, T-3 h], [T-3 h, T-12 h], and [T-12 h, T-24 h]. In the literature, there is no universal definition of the critical time intervals in diabetes management. The selected intervals are based on expert medical opinion, and translate important time periods, namely the pre-meal, pre-insulin administration, or the average duration of the influence of an exercise or physical exertion on glycaemia values. Later time-intervals were deemed unnecessary, as their value range consisted of a single value type. Glycaemia-based features are associated with the same range of intervals excluding the interval [T, T-30min], as this interval would contain data too close to the values to be classified or predicted. The final data set is composed of 98 features, represented in Fig. 1. In it, each row represents a specific feature with the corresponding time ranges that it has defined. For example S. TIR (Sensor Time In Range) is measured on the [T-30min, T-1 h], [T-1h, T-3 h], [T-3 h, T-12 h], and [T-12 h, T-24 h] time ranges. In the figure *S.* indicates a feature from a Sensor, whereas *F.* is

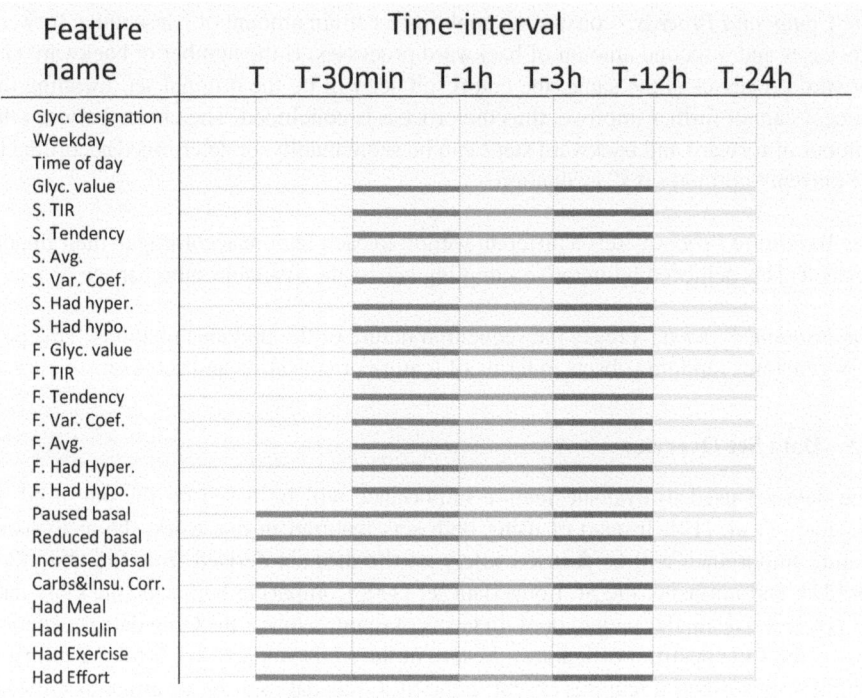

Fig. 1. Ohio-based data set's feature space.

from a measure with a finger-prick. *Glyc.* means glycaemia, *Var. Coef.* is the variance coefficient, *Carbs&Insu. Corr.* means the correlation between the consumed carbohydrates and insulin intake.

The data set is, by default, imbalanced. To correct this, the set was balanced using the most appropriated balancing approach for this set: a joint use of SMOTE and ENN [19]. In Figs. 2 and 3 it is possible to perceive the impact of the balancing approach. The most inner circle represents the number of hypoglycaemias by the radius of the sector. The middle annulus represents the number of euglycaemias, and the outer annulus the number of hyperglycaemias.

2.4 Feature Importance Implementation

To calculate feature importance, it is necessary to first choose a model to run the different tests. Considering the Gini importance requirements, the most appropriate approach would be to use a tree-based model. As all tests should be executed in an equal environment, the model chosen to calculate Gini importance will also be used for the remaining tests. Two tree-based models were considered:

(i) Decision tree is a supervised data mining learning method, shaped as a tree. It maps available outcomes in a series of possible decisions. This non-parametric

The Impact of Feature Selection on Balancing, Based on Diabetes Data   131

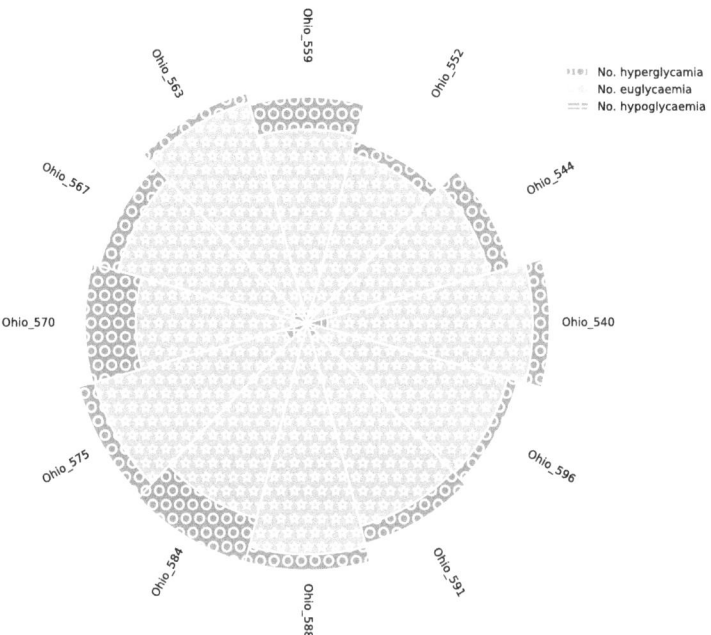

Fig. 2. Ohio's data set glycaemia statistics before balancing.

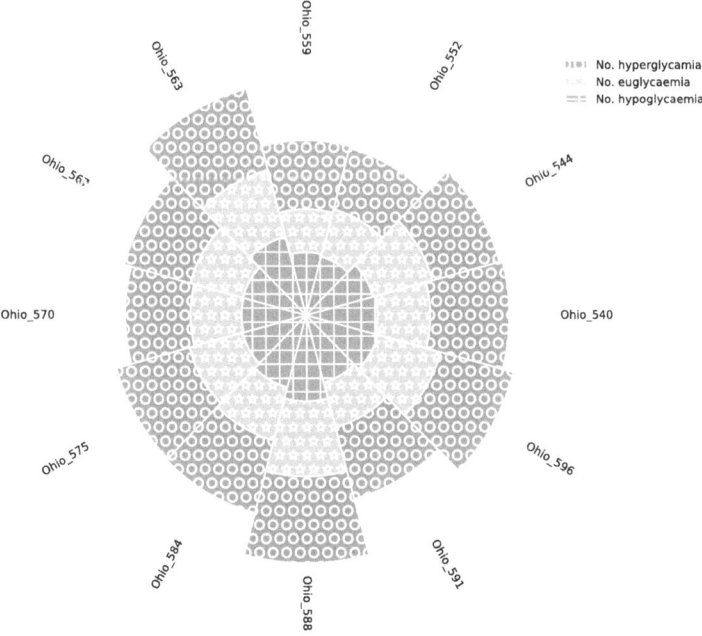

Fig. 3. Ohio's data set glycaemia statistics after balancing.

method is normally used for classification and regression, but it can also be used for the study of feature importance [9,11,28].

(ii) Random forest is an ensemble learning method, commonly used for classification and regression. This method consists of a collection of decision trees. The decisions made by the random forest method are obtained through majority vote of the trees that constitute the model. It utilises bagging and feature randomness to create uncorrelated sets of decision trees. Feature randomness guarantees low correlation amidst decision trees [5].

Contrary to decision trees, the random forest method, when composed of a robust number of trees, has a reduced risk of over-fitting. As decision trees are frequently associated with over-fitting, it was decided to instead use random forest as the model for the study of feature importance.

Metrics. The analysis of a model's performance can be accessed through a confusion matrix. A confusion matrix encompasses the results of the relation between the model predictions and the true values. This matrix is composed of: the true positives (TP), values that were correctly predicted as the positive class; the true negatives (TN), values that were correctly predicted as the negative class; the false positives (FP), values that were wrongly predicted as the positive class; and the false negatives (FN), values that were incorrectly predicted as the negative class. Considering that the model will have three possible classifications, the resulting confusion matrix will be composed of three rows and three columns. Associated to the confusion matrix are a number of metrics that describe the model's performance from different perspectives.

– Accuracy is the ratio of correct predictions to total predictions made.
$$Accuracy = \frac{TP}{Total predictions}$$

– Sensitivity (true positive rate) reflects the model's ability to correctly identify positive cases.
$$Sensitivity = \frac{TP}{TP + FN}$$

– Specificity (true negative rate) reflects the model's ability to detect negative cases.
$$Specificity = \frac{TN}{TN + FP}$$

– Precision is a metric that quantifies the number of correct positive predictions over all positive predicted values.
$$Precision = \frac{T_p}{(T_p + F_p)}$$

– Recall quantifies the number of correct positive predictions over all possible positive predictions.
$$Recall = \frac{T_p}{(T_p + F_n)}$$

- The F-Measure (Fβ) [26] conjugates the precision and the recall in a single metric, considering their harmonic mean. Rather than focusing on accuracy, the Fβ focuses on the positive class, which, in an imbalanced data set, has a greater impact than accuracy. Higher Fβ values are associated with a better performance of the model.

$$F\beta = \frac{(1+\beta)^2 * precision * recall}{\beta^2 * recall + precision}$$

  β represents the relative weight given to precision in respect to recall [4]. The F1-score, one of the most known and used metrics, attributes the same importance to precision as well as to recall.
- The Geometric Mean (G-Mean) combines sensitivity and specificity in a single metric [1]. It calculates the geometric mean of the positive and negative class, trying to maximise both, whilst maintaining a balance [4, 14].

$$G\text{-}Mean = \sqrt{Sensitivity * Specificity}$$

- The Receiver Operating Characteristic (ROC) curve [8] enables a visual representation of the compromise between benefits and costs, along different threshold levels.
- Precision-recall curves are a form of ROC curve for the context of precision and recall for binary classification. In the case of multi-class, this method has to be adapted. Each class has to be evaluated separately against the other classes. A perfect model will maximise both the precision and the recall throughout different thresholds, resulting in a higher area under the curve. Precision-recall curves are recommended for substantially imbalanced data sets [3, 4].
- The Average Precision is the weighted mean of precision values, achieved at different thresholds of the precision-recall curve, with the increase in recall from the previous threshold as weight. This metric can be represented as shown in equation 2.4, where (P_n) and (R_n) are the precision and recall at the nth threshold, respectively.

$$\text{``}AveragePrecision\text{''} = \sum_{n}(R_n - R_{n-1})P_n$$

Although all the referred measures are valid evaluation metrics, in the context of imbalanced data sets, the F1-score and precision-recall are regarded as the most appropriate for imbalanced data sets. In the context of this study, as a single value metric is required to properly rank feature importance approaches, the F1-score was chosen. In the study of diabetes management, the states of hypoglycaemia and hyperglycaemia take precedence over the euglycaemia states (normal glycaemia values). To measure the model's performance whilst maintaining focus on these states, three F1-scores were calculated: one for hypoglycaemia, one for hyperglycaemia, and one for non-euglycaemia. The weighted average of the three F1-scores was calculated as a final score. The weight of each classification is inversely related to their representation on the test data set, meaning that hypoglycaemia should have a heavier weight on the score. Note that whilst the model's training set is balanced, the test set is not.

2.5 Re-Evaluating the Balancing Methods

The impact of a balancing approach to a set exhibits variances reliant on the data available. Therefore, it is not possible to choose beforehand the best balancing approach. The choice of approach often falls on personal preference or on uncovering the best method through brute force.

Once an optimal feature space is achieved, it could be reasoned that, whilst the remaining features contain the same data values, the correlation between features changed, thus the resulting data set is different. This fact may also imply that the balancing approach that was once the best, may now be subpar. If this assumption is correct, it indicates that, when granted a superior feature space, it is relevant to re-evaluate the chosen balancing approach.

In this context, a re-evaluation of the conclusions by [19] on the Ohio data set will be conducted using an optimal feature set. The evaluation will use the same methodology as in [19]. Random forest will be used as the classification model, and F1 as the evaluation metric.

3 Feature Importance Results

To understand the role of each feature and reach an optimised feature set, both individual feature importance and optimal set search were performed. These methods will allow the understanding of the main contributors to the model's decision and achieve a superior feature set that will enhance the model's performance.

3.1 Individual Feature Study Results

The feature individual score refers to the feature's influence in the corresponding data set. Considering that the Ohio data set is composed of 12 patients, it is necessary to unify the different scores in a single metric. For these tests, the individual importance of each feature was calculated for each patient. The average feature value is selected to represent the overall feature importance among all patients. The standard deviation can be seen as the consensus among patients on the feature's value.

Gini Results. The Gini evaluation places as the five most important features: sensor-based time in range, the latest glycaemia value, the glycaemia average, the existence of previous hyperglycaemia and the glycaemia tendency within the time interval of the last 30 min to one hour. All of these features are glycaemia-based. The purpose of the study of diabetes is to either prevent it, or assist patients in their management of diabetes. This can be achieved in multiple manners. Having access to features that represent concrete patient actions can be used to advise patients on how to improve their diabetes-management. Generally glycaemia-based features do not offer a good explanation for why a hypo or hyperglycaemia occurred as they represent a glycaemia state. There is a correlation between glycaemia tendency and the future value of glycaemia (hyper, hypo or euglycaemia), but this connection alone is not sufficient to explain to the patient why the hyper or hypo occurred: was the current hypoglycaemia state due to an exercise without food compensation?, was the current hyperglycaemia due to an insufficient insulin intake after a meal? These features are good for occurrence detection, but do not explain the behaviours that led to it. Of the top five features, the exception is the existence of a recent hyperglycaemia. This feature provides a particular plausible cause that can be used to advise the patient of for example a hypoglycaemia.

Figure 4 illustrates the results obtained, detailing the importance of the time ranges for each feature. The inner circle represents the overall feature importance, given by the length of the arc. The outer annulus represents the importance of the specific time range for that feature.

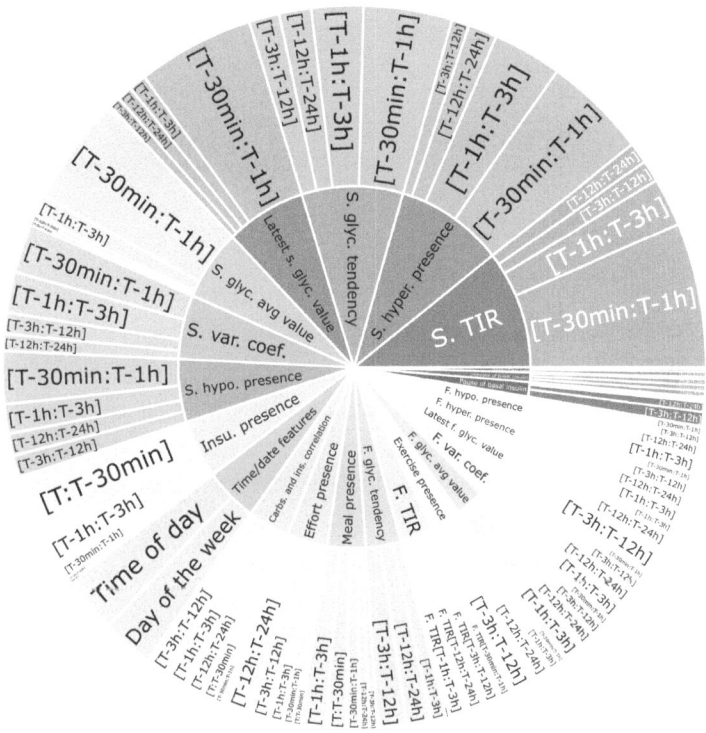

Fig. 4. Gini importance results.

The five worse features, according to the average score, were all related to manual alterations of the basal insulin. These features could indicate a reasonable cause for hyper and hypoglycaemia. The fact that they are so lowly ranked indicates that, for the method, these feature are not correlated with hypo or hyperglycaemia states. These manual alterations most certainly were prescribed by an medical expert and followed correctly. The rationale is that if the adjustment was correct the glycaemia values will tend to be normal. Thus, the detection of hypo or hyperglycaemia will not be influenced by the adjustments on the basal insulin.

MDA Results. The MDA evaluation's top five scoring features were the last glycaemia value, the glycaemia average, the occurrence of hyperglycaemia, the glycaemia time-in-range in the 30 min to one hour interval, and the finger-based glycaemia average in the last one to three hours. The worse five features, according to the MDA evaluation, were the existence of insulin, finger-based variation coefficient in the one to three hour time interval, the correlation between insulin and meals, and the existence of finger-based hyperglycaemia in the 12 to 24 h time interval, and the time of day. The representation of the obtained results is displayed on Fig. 5. It uses the same representation as in Fig. 4.

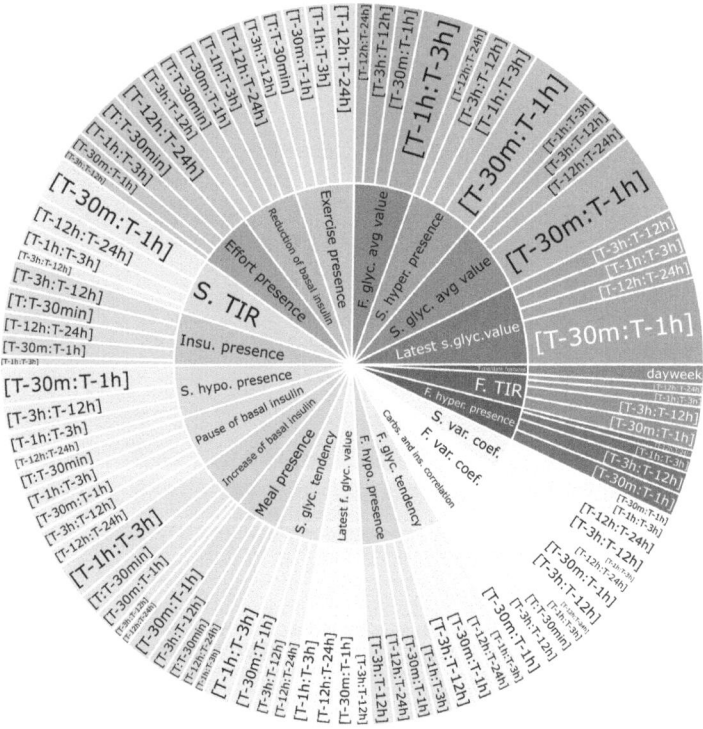

Fig. 5. MDA importance results.

Although the top five features are very similar to the Gini evaluation, the worse scoring features are distinct. The MDA table shows that, in terms of MDA scores, manual changes to the basal insulin can be significant.

Forward Drop Feature Search Results. The forward drop column search isolates the feature importance by evaluating the before and the aftermath results of dropping a certain feature. The evaluation metric used in this test was the F1-score. The feature's importance, in this test, is determined by the difference in value between the baseline (set with the feature) and the set without the feature. A score close or equal to zero, shows that the dropped feature does not have any impact on the model. A score greater than zero means that the evaluation of the data set without the selected feature obtained a worse score than when it was included, thus the referred feature is relevant. On the other hand if the score is negative, then the set without the selected feature performs better than the baseline, meaning the feature is deemed prejudicial. The representation of the obtained results is displayed on Fig. 6. As the results of this approach process contains negative values, the values had to be normalised to then be represented in this graphic form.

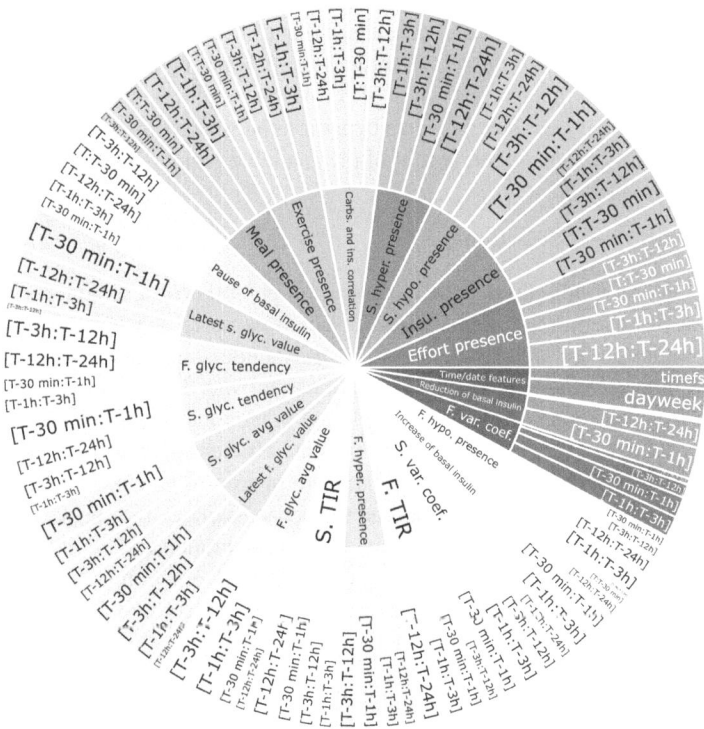

Fig. 6. Drop feature results.

The results obtained do not point to a clear set of important features. The feature space is composed by values very close to zero. One feature has a zero score (Day of the week). A great majority of values received a negative difference score. The feature set size can justify the low score range. In this set no feature has a substantial participation, instead all the features have small contributions.

In this test, the features' standard deviation was higher than their average score. This proves that each patient is unique in respect to feature importance. Although some features may be important for a patient, regarding the patient population, the feature's importance is diminished. Therefore, only the common most important features will receive a positive score.

The effort feature within the 12 to 24 h interval received the best individual score (0.91 percentile point increase). The minimum score obtained was -0.62 and maximum of 4.84 percentile points. It should be noted that only six of the 12 patients have records of effort.

Congruent with the previous results, the last available sensor-based glycaemia value, within the [T-30 min, T-1 h] time interval, was the second better scoring feature. This feature's importance is attested not only by its positive score, and by its consistent appearance among the top features in every individual importance feature test.

The remaining features that compose the top 5 best features were the presence of hypoglycaemia, the sensor-based tendency and average glycaemia value.

The record's weekday obtained an average score of zero. It should be noted that, for some patients, the day of the week feature was relevant. Nonetheless, the maximum percentile increase by this feature was 1.74. From this result, it is possible to infer that some patients do have a tendency to have hypo or hyperglycaemia in certain days of the week, although this is not a general trait of the available patient population.

3.2 Best Feature Set Selection

Individual feature results do not fully convey the potential of a feature in a set. Two features can be insignificant while isolated, albeit essential when together to obtain a correct prediction and/or classification. To fully understand the scope of each features' importance, the best feature set for each patient was determined. Three methods were used: forward search, backward search and branch and bound. Whilst sequential searches do not return the optimal sub-set, they are efficient procedures able to remove redundant features. Furthermore, if these sets are proven to be equal or similar to the optimal feature set, it is plausible to assume the non-existence of synergy between non-sequential features. As previously mentioned, although branch and bound is capable of calculating the optimal feature set, its computing cost may render it unfeasible in a real-life context. Differing from individual importance, the selection of the best feature set does not offer a tangible score. For this reason, it is not possible to conclude an average score for each feature.

To evaluate the significance of the obtained feature set, the best feature set F1-score will be compared to its baseline. Additionally, the features that compose the optimal set, will be ranked by "popular vote". Each patient will have an optimal feature set and the features present in this set will each receive a "vote". These votes rank the different features. The more votes a feature has, the more important it is. It is challenging to establish a clear threshold that divides essential from non-essential features. The focus of the feature importance study is to reach a sub-set with optimal characteristics to the majority of patients. Therefore, features with a number of votes less or equal to six (half the number of patients), should not be considered. It should be noted that some features are exclusive to a smaller patient sub set. In this case, if the features are deemed important, but do not reach a majority of patients, they should be considered for individual evaluation.

To determine the optimal feature set, three tests were conducted:

Sequential Forward Search Results. This test starts with an empty set and added, at each iteration, the best scoring feature; every other feature not yet in the set is included, and the score calculated for the set. The process stopped when the best available feature to be added had a score that was worse than the previous state. This process was executed for each patient. In the end, to get the best common features, the voting process was applied.

The average F1-score using this method was 60.76% with a standard deviation of 10.53%. This method generated for all patients reduced feature sets. On average the patients "optimal sets" were composed of three features, with a maximum of seven features and a minimum of a single feature. The reduced feature spaces produced by this method do not allow a significant overlap of common features among patients.

Sequential Backward Search Results. Although similar to the previous process, the backward search begins with a full set of features. Sequentially, the worst feature of the set is removed until no more features can be removed. The process is halted if the set containing the feature to be removed performs better than the set without the feature.

The average F1-score using this method was 64.03% with a standard deviation of 9.29%. This method achieved an average score four percentile points above the forward search, and a minor standard deviation. Although this approach's performance appears to be better than the previous, its standard deviation is still unsatisfactory.

This method, for every patient, reached a plateau in a very early stage. On average each patient subtracted two features. The resulting common feature space is composed by every feature available.

Branch and Bound Search Results. This method is capable of analysing the full spectrum of feature set possibilities. Consequently, this method is able to uncover an optimal solution. The method's caveat is its complexity, which is exponential in the worst case [34]. Although a set of irrelevant features was removed, the average number of features each data set contains remains around 90. Despite reducing from the 147 features from the original, this feature space still requires great computational resources that are not available to the project. With a sufficient time-frame, this method could be successfully ran. Unfortunately, considering the goal of advising patients, the time-frame needed would not be realistically feasible.

Considering the complexity of this test, and the defined objectives, a normal individual feature study is not possible. Instead, the branch and bound method was applied to feature groups. Each feature belongs to a single group, contrary to the previous sequential group test where features could be represented in more than one group. A total of 23 groups were defined, one for each different data aspect. By scaling down the feature set to 23, the process of branch and bound becomes feasible within a reasonable time-frame. The obtained results are shown in Fig. 7.

The branch and bound average F1-score was 67.10% with a standard deviation of 9.32%. This method, although altered to work with feature groups instead of single features, achieved a significantly better performance than the previous methods. The standard deviation continues to be substantial, thus supporting the notion that, given

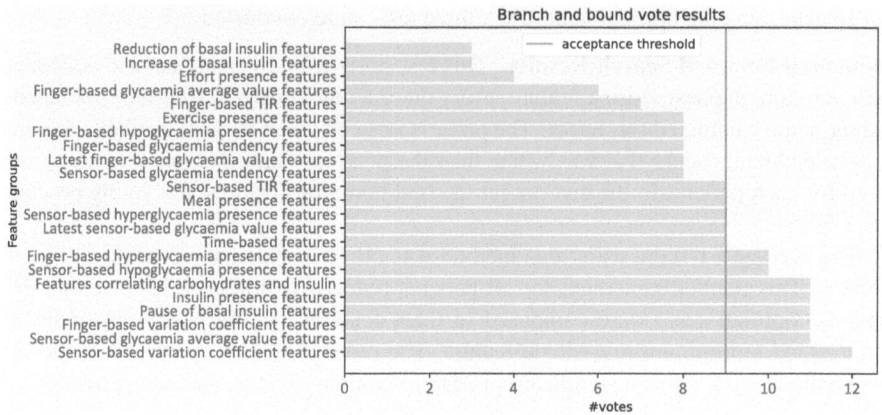

Fig. 7. Branch and bound results.

how diverse the patients are, it is not possible to reach a general yet optimal feature set for all patients. All existing feature groups received votes, which implies that every feature group holds a degree of relative importance.

The features' groups that are most representative of the majority of patients (75% or more) were the Sensor-based variation coefficient features, the Sensor-based glycaemia average value features, the Finger-based variation coefficient features, the Pause of basal insulin features, the Insulin presence features, the Features correlating carbohydrates and insulin, the Sensor-based hypoglycaemia presence features, the Finger-based hyperglycaemia presence features, the Time-based features, the Latest sensor-based glycaemia value features, the Sensor-based hyperglycaemia presence features, the Meal presence features, and the Sensor-based TIR features. The Increase of basal insulin features, and Exercise presence features feature groups reach a relative 75% majority, considering only the patient population with these records. Although these feature groups will not be incorporated into the branch and bound result, they can be considered in other, more individual, approaches. The branch and bound most representative set, embodies the essential features for all patients. Nonetheless, features external to this set such as Increase of basal insulin features, and Exercise presence features, can be used for specific patient subgroups to enhance performance.

The feature importance results point to a possible need to personalise the study of the patient's data. Overall, the results standard deviation remained high, showing diversity within the patient set. Considering the results, it is important to understand how granular the patient heterogeneity is. This analysis will help determine whether patients can be grouped together or if it is necessary to conduct an individual study for each patient.

4 Re-evaluation of the Balancing Approaches

The proposed optimal set could not be reached due to time and computational constraints. Nevertheless, it was possible to attain a superior feature space, capable of enhancing the model's performance. Despite its sub-optimal nature, the attained feature space represents a superior variant of the full set. It is thus assumed that the superior version of the set will lead to an enhanced model performance. If optimal, further performance improvement should be expected. Regardless, the focal point of this work is not pure performance, but to perceive if the balancing approaches' impact remains consistent regardless of the number of features. Figure 8 displays the difference in performance using the full feature space and the better feature set that was achieved in this work. It should be noted that the F1 score values range from 0 to 1. Thus, on the right of the figure, we have the F1 score after the balancing approach mentioned was applied using the full feature set for each of hypo, hyperglycaemia and non-euglycaemia. On the left, we have the F1 score after balancing using only the calculated best feature set.

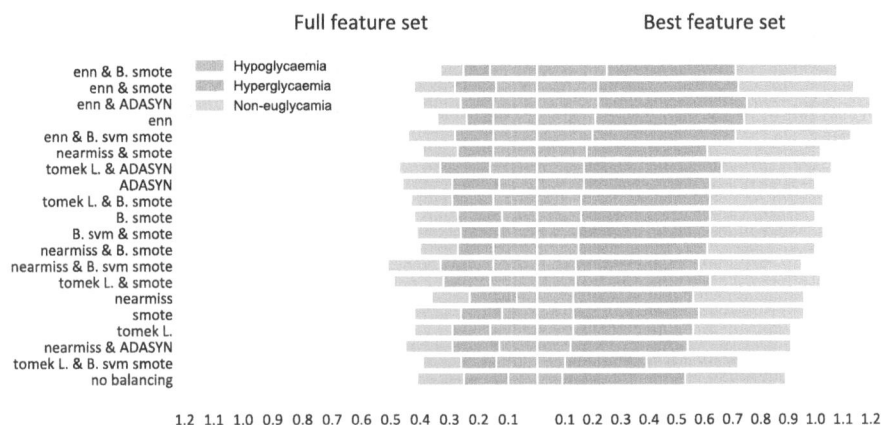

Fig. 8. Comparison of the F1 impact of balancing using a full set and the best feature set.

A visible consequence of applying feature importance is, as expected, the overall increase in F1 score. Concerning the best approaches, the use of ENN and SMOTE continue to be among the top approaches. Interestingly, ENN as a sole approach, is the best scoring approach (using the better feature set), thus evidencing the importance of this under-sampling method. Previously, with the availability of the full feature space, ENN was ranked as the fourth-best approach. ENN and ADASYN was ranked as the second-best approach, and, in third place, appears ENN and SMOTE. The improvement in performance is divided in three classes: hypoglycaemia, hyperglycaemia and non-euglycaemia. Of the three classes, hypoglycaemia was the least impacted by using the best feature set. On the other hand, the hyperglycaemia and non-euglycaemia classes reached substantial performance gains.

Comparing the array of approaches, using the best feature set, it appears that the difference in performance is substantial. To assert the value of each approach, the partial performance gains/losses have to be individually considered. Summing partial performance gains can lead to inaccurate conclusions. The performance gains/losses of each approach, in respect to hypo, hyper, and non-euglycaemia, are shown in Fig. 9. The figure shows the increase (positive value on the graph) or decrease (negative value on the graph) on the F1 score with the best feature set after applying each balancing approach.

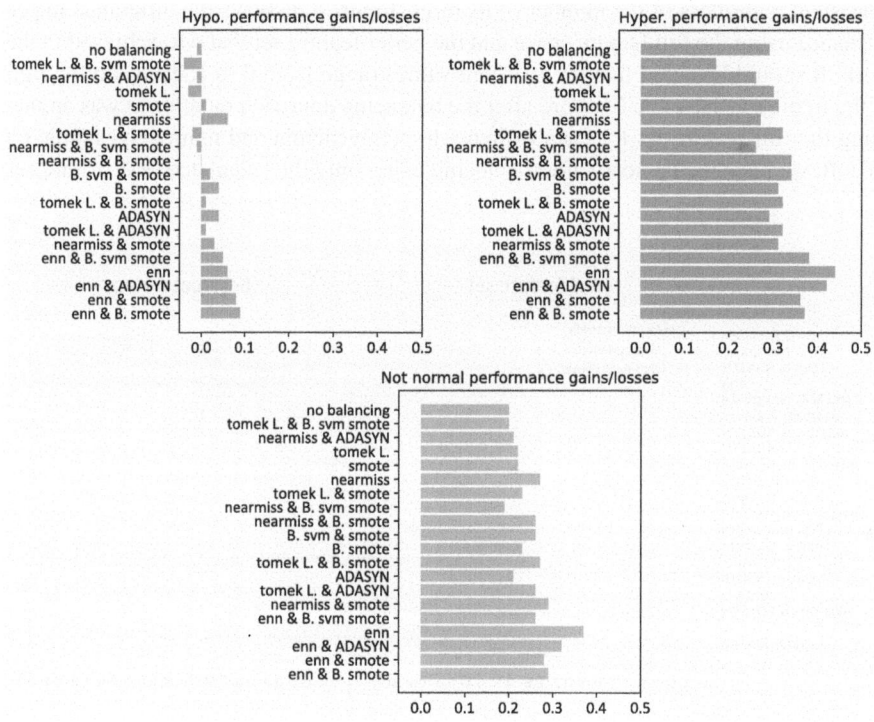

Fig. 9. Performance difference for each glycaemia aspect.

The disparities in performance shown in Fig. 9, indicate hypoglycaemia as the primary distinguishing factor. As for hyperglycaemia and non-euglycaemia, the overall differences are significant, but similar among balancing approaches. Considering the previous best balancing approach (ENN and SMOTE) and the now best scoring approach (ENN), it is not clear which is the best approach. With regard to hypoglycaemia, ENN and SMOTE have a score two percentile points better than the ENN approach. With respect to hyper and non-euglycaemia, the ENN approach is better 6 and 4 percentile points respectively. In terms of overall performance, it is not possible to conclude which approach is superior. This assumption is dependent on the class to be prioritised. Additionally, The disparity in performance between the two approaches may not be considered significant.

Analysing the results, it is possible to affirm that feature importance has an effect on the impact of the balancing approach. Although in this concrete case, the difference in performance may not be considered as significant, it is still existent. It is possible to speculate that in other types of data this disparity may be greater and significant, thus it may be prudent to re-evaluate the balancing approach after reaching a superior feature space.

5 Conclusion

Diabetes data is scarce and has a strong imbalance due to the over-representation of euglycaemia values. Although the majority of data sets, related to diabetes, are solely composed by glycaemia values, diabetes management is composed by a series of factors and glycaemia metrics. Actions, such as meals, insulin intake, exercise, and efforts, have a significant impact on glycaemia. When these factors, and other indicators, are considered, the resulting data set may contain an excessive number of features. Feature importance allows a better understanding of the impact of each feature in the model's conclusion. Additionally, feature importance may provide a sub-set of optimal features, enhancing performance, and reducing computational costs.

In terms of individual feature evaluation approaches, the drop feature method is to be preferred. MDI and MDA could be considered, if the computational overhead associated to the drop feature method is excessive. Relative to the study of the optimal feature set, the forward and backward search approaches are sub-par and returned very poor results. The greedy nature of these methods limits the method's progression beyond an early stage, consequently inhibiting the discovery of potentially superior subsets. The branch-and-bound method is able to reach this optimal set, albeit it requires a heavy computational effort. In this work, it was not possible to fully execute branch-and-bound, due to computational and time limitations. To obtain meaningful results, it was necessary to introduce adaptations to the method, namely the creation of feature groups to decrease the number of available features.

The use of a better feature set, even if not optimal, influenced the performance of the balancing methods. In the case of the Ohio data set, the difference in performance was not substantial. Nonetheless, the existence of a differential proves that there may exist a case where the gap in performance may be sufficient to consider a different balancing approach.

References

1. Akosa, J.S.: Predictive accuracy : a misleading performance measure for highly imbalanced data (2017)
2. Babai, L.: Monte-carlo algorithms in graph isomorphism testing. Université tde Montréal Technical Report, DMS pp. 79–10 (1979). https://www.bibsonomy.org/bibtex/28e63f01a447ec6747b2ac926d83b7771/pcbouman
3. Branco, P., Torgo, L., Ribeiro, R.: A survey of predictive modelling under imbalanced distributions (2015). https://doi.org/10.48550/ARXIV.1505.01658
4. Branco, P., Torgo, L., Ribeiro, R.P.: A survey of predictive modeling on imbalanced domains. ACM Comput. Surv. **49**(2) (aug 2016). https://doi.org/10.1145/2907070
5. Breiman, L.: Random forests. Mach. Learn. **45**(1), 5–32 (2001). https://doi.org/10.1023/A:1010933404324

6. Breiman, L.: Manual on setting up, using, and understanding random forests v3.1 (Jan 2002). https://www.stat.berkeley.edu/~breiman/Using_random_forests_V3.1.pdf. Accessed 12 Sept 2022
7. Doak, J.: An evaluation of feature selection methodsand their application to computer security. UC Davis: College of Engineering (1992). Retrieved on 31/03/2023 .https://escholarship.org/uc/item/2jf918dh
8. Egan, J.P.: Signal detection theory and roc analysis (1975)
9. Fan, W., Liu, K., Liu, H., Ge, Y., Xiong, H., Fu, Y.: Interactive reinforcement learning for feature selection with decision tree in the loop. IEEE Trans. Knowl. Data Eng. **35**(2), 1624–1636 (2023). https://doi.org/10.1109/TKDE.2021.3102120
10. Federation, I.D.: Idf diabetes atlas, 9th edn. brussels (2019). https://www.diabetesatlas.org. Accessed 19 July 2021
11. Grabczewski, K., Jankowski, N.: Feature selection with decision tree criterion. In: Fifth International Conference on Hybrid Intelligent Systems (HIS'05), pp. 6 pp.– (2005). https://doi.org/10.1109/ICHIS.2005.43
12. Guyon, I., Elisseeff, A.: An introduction to variable and feature selection. J. Mach. Learn. Res. **3**(null), 1157-1182 (mar 2003)
13. Kahn, M.: Diabetes. UCI Machine Learning Repository. https://doi.org/10.24432/C5T59G
14. Kubat, M., Holte, R.C., Matwin, S.: Machine learning for the detection of oil spills in satellite radar images. Mach. Learn. **30**(2/3), 195–215 (1998). https://doi.org/10.1023/a:1007452223027
15. Kumar, V.: Feature selection: A literature review. Smart Comput. Rev. **4**(3) (Jun 2014). https://doi.org/10.6029/smartcr.2014.03.007
16. Li, D., Liu, C., Hu, S.C.: A learning method for the class imbalance problem with medical data sets. Comput. Biol. Med. **40**(5), 509–518 (2010). https://doi.org/10.1016/j.compbiomed.2010.03.005
17. Li, J., et al.: Feature selection. ACM Comput. Surv. **50**(6), 1–45 (2017). https://doi.org/10.1145/3136625
18. Li, J.: Feature selection. ACM Comput. Surv. **50**(6), 1–45 (2018). https://doi.org/10.1145/3136625
19. Machado, D., Costa, V., Brandão, P.: Using balancing methods to improve glycaemia-based data mining. In: Proceedings of the 16th International Joint Conference on Biomedical Engineering Systems and Technologies. SCITEPRESS - Science and Technology Publications (2023). https://doi.org/10.5220/0011797100003414
20. Machado, D., Costa, V.S., Brandão, P.: Impact of the glycaemic sampling method in diabetes data mining. In: 2022 IEEE Symposium on Computers and Communications (ISCC), pp. 1–6 (2022). https://doi.org/10.1109/ISCC55528.2022.9912822
21. Marling, C., Bunescu, R.C.: The OhioT1DM dataset for blood glucose level prediction: Update 2020. In: Bach, K., Bunescu, R.C., Marling, C., Wiratunga, N. (eds.) Proceedings of the 5th International Workshop on Knowledge Discovery in Healthcare Data co-located with 24th European Conference on Artificial Intelligence, KDH@ECAI 2020, Santiago de Compostela, Spain & Virtually, August 29-30, 2020. CEUR Workshop Proceedings, vol. 2675, pp. 71–74. CEUR-WS.org (2020). http://ceur-ws.org/Vol-2675/paper11.pdf
22. Molina, L., Belanche, L., Nebot, A.: Feature selection algorithms: a survey and experimental evaluation. In: 2002 IEEE International Conference on Data Mining, 2002. Proceedings., pp. 306–313 (2002). https://doi.org/10.1109/ICDM.2002.1183917
23. Mouri, M., Badireddy, M.: Hyperglycemia. StatPearls [Internet] (Jan 2021). https://www.ncbi.nlm.nih.gov/books/NBK430900/. [Updated 2021 May 10]
24. Narendra, F.: A branch and bound algorithm for feature subset selection. IEEE Trans. Comput. **C-26**(9), 917–922 (1977). https://doi.org/10.1109/TC.1977.1674939

25. Raval, K.M.: Data mining techniques. Int. J. Adv. Res. Comput. Sci. Softw. Eng. **2**(10) (2012)
26. Rijsbergen, C.J.V.: Information Retrieval, 2nd edn. Butterworth-Heinemann, USA (1979)
27. Scornet, E.: Trees, forests, and impurity-based variable importance. arXiv (Jan 2020). https://doi.org/10.48550/arXiv.2001.04295
28. Scornet, E.: Trees, forests, and impurity-based variable importance in regression. Ann. Inst. Henri Poincaré Probab. Stat. **59**(1), 21–52 (2023). https://doi.org/10.1214/21-AIHP1240
29. Seery, C.: Diabetes complications. guide on diabetes.co.uk (2019). https://www.diabetes.co.uk/diabetes-complications/diabetes-complications.html, accessed on: 20/07/2021
30. Seery, C.: Short term complications. guide on diabetes.co.uk (2019). https://www.diabetes.co.uk/diabetes-complications/short-term-complications.html. Accessed 20 July 2021
31. Shukla, D., Patel, S.B., Sen, A.K.: A literature review in health informatics using data mining techniques. Int. J. Softw. Hardw. Res. Eng. **2**(2), 123–129 (2014)
32. Strobl, C., Boulesteix, A.L., Kneib, T., Augustin, T., Zeileis, A.: Conditional variable importance for random forests. BMC Bioinf. **9**(1), 1–11 (2008). https://doi.org/10.1186/1471-2105-9-307
33. Terence, P., Kerem, T., Christopher, C., Jeremy, H.: Beware Default Random Forest Importances (Jun 2020). https://explained.ai/rf-importance/index.html. Accessed 12 Sept 2022
34. Thakoor, N., Devarajan, V., Gao, J.: Computation complexity of branch-and-bound model selection. In: 2009 IEEE 12th International Conference on Computer Vision. IEEE (Sep 2009). https://doi.org/10.1109/iccv.2009.5459420
35. Wojtas, M., Chen, K.: Feature importance ranking for deep learning (2020). https://doi.org/10.48550/ARXIV.2010.08973

Author Index

A
Aguila, Maria Eliza R. 107
Altaf, Muahammad Awais Bin 40
Anlacan, Veeda Michelle M. 107
Apuya, Romuel Aloizeus Z. 107
Araujo, Helder 1

B
Bain, Michael 60
Barker, Christopher 60
Brandão, Pedro 125

C
Caro, Jaime D. L. 107
Costa, Vítor Santos 125

G
Galecio, Bryan Andrei C. 107
Good, Norm 60

H
Hartwig, Mattis 84

I
Ismail, Iman A. 24

J
Jamora, Roland Dominic G. 107

K
Kamavuako, Ernest N. 24
Kemp, James 60
Khan, Gul Hameed 40
Khan, Nadeem Ahmad 40
Kirsten, Toralf 84

M
Machado, Diogo 125

O
Oliveira, Marina 1

P
Panganiban, Angelo Cedric F. 107

S
Saadeh, Wala 40
Salido, Isabel Teresa O. 107

T
Tee, Cherica A. 107
Tee, Michael L. 107

W
Winter, Alexander 84

SPRINGER NATURE

GPSR Compliance

The European Union's (EU) General Product Safety Regulation (GPSR) is a set of rules that requires consumer products to be safe and our obligations to ensure this.

If you have any concerns about our products, you can contact us on ProductSafety@springernature.com

In case Publisher is established outside the EU, the EU authorized representative is:

Springer Nature Customer Service Center GmbH
Europaplatz 3
69115 Heidelberg, Germany

The manufacturer's authorised representative in the EU is Springer Nature Customer Service Centre GmbH, Europaplatz 3, 69115 Heidelberg, Germany. If you have any concerns regarding our products, please contact ProductSafety@springernature.com

Printed and bound by CPI Group (UK) Ltd, Croydon, CR0 4YY

26/03/2026

02078975-0005